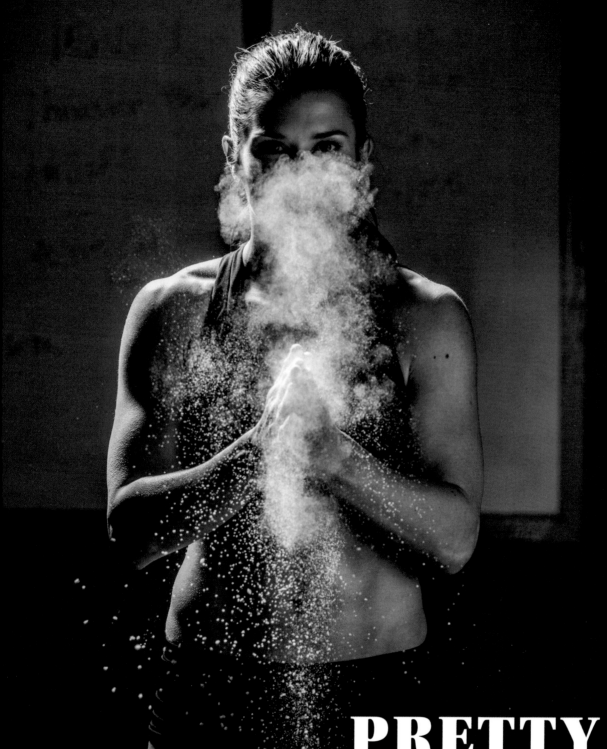

PRETTY
INTENSE

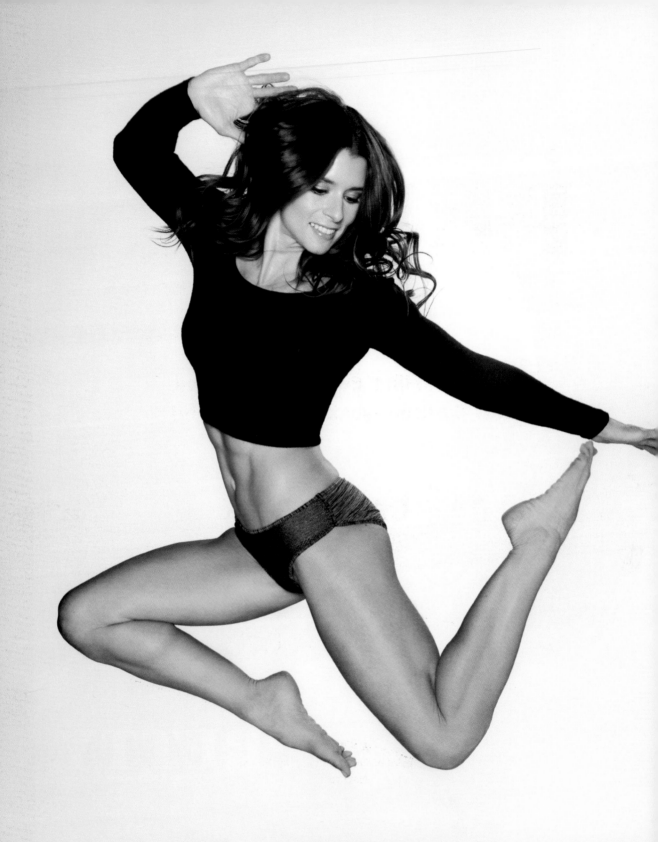

PRETTY INTENSE

The 90-Day Mind, Body and Food Plan
That Will Absolutely Change Your Life!

DANICA PATRICK
with Stephen Perrine

AVERY
an imprint of Penguin Random House
New York

AVERY

An imprint of Penguin Random House LLC
375 Hudson Street
New York, New York 10014

Most Avery books are available at special quantity discounts for bulk
purchase for sales promotions, premiums, fund-raising, and educational
needs. Special books or book excerpts also can be created to fit specific needs.
For details, write SpecialMarkets@penguinrandomhouse.com.

Library of Congress Cataloging-in-Publication Data

Names: Patrick, Danica, 1982- author.
Title: Pretty intense : the 90-day mind, body and food plan that will
    absolutely change your life! / by Danica Patrick with Stephen Perrine.
Description: New York : Avery, an imprint of Penguin Random House,
    [2018] | Includes bibliographical references and index.
Identifiers: LCCN 2017031129| ISBN 9780735216563 (hardback) |
    ISBN 9780735216570 (epub)
Subjects: LCSH: Reducing exercises. | Reducing diets. | Physical fitness. |
    Weight loss. | BISAC: HEALTH & FITNESS / Vitamins. | COOKING /
    Health & Healing / General.
Classification: LCC RA781.6 .P38 2018 | DDC 613.7—dc23 LC record
    available at https://lccn.loc.gov/2017031129

p.   cm.

Printed in the United States of America
0 9 8 7 6 5 4 3 2 1

Book design by Ashley Tucker

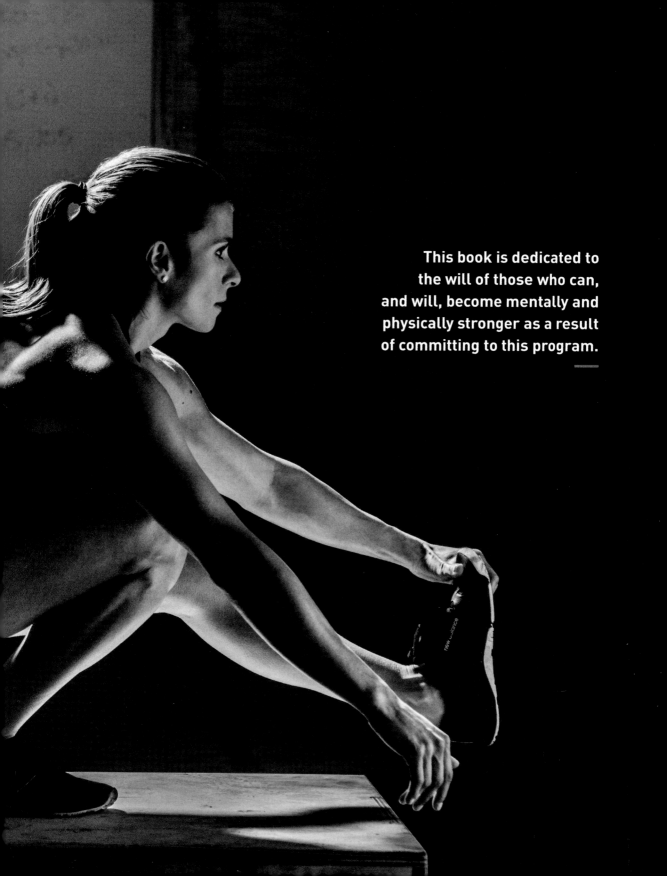

This book is dedicated to the will of those who can, and will, become mentally and physically stronger as a result of committing to this program.

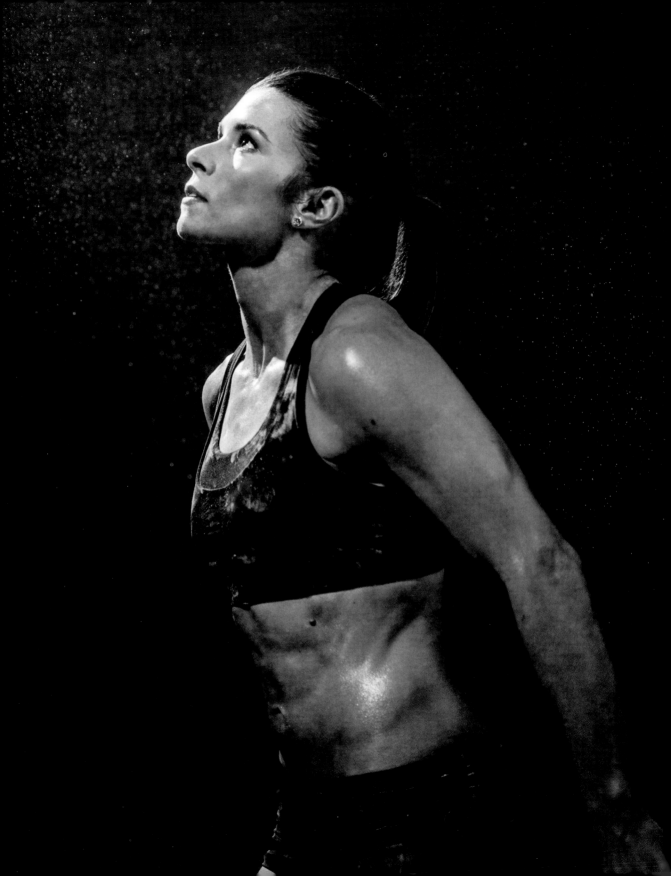

People say I'm pretty intense.

    Wouldn't it be cool if "pretty intense" was the way they talked about you, too?

If they described your body, your mind, your career, the way you live your entire life, as "pretty intense"? If you looked and felt the way you've always dreamed of being—lean, strong, and confident? If you had the ability to attack and achieve your physical and mental goals with such self-empowerment that no one could stand in your way?

That's what *Pretty Intense* will give you: It's a high-intensity diet, fitness, and mental-conditioning program for people who want to live an intense and successful life. It will reshape your body, calm your mind, and set you on the path to achieving your life's greatest goals.

And it will be more fun than you ever imagined.

With the *Pretty Intense* program, I will show you how to eat and how to exercise to achieve a lean, strong, sculpted body while taking control of your health, your weight, and your life. But more important, I will give you the tools you need to become the person you want to be—to overcome negativity and self-doubt, to stay motivated and strong, and to prove to yourself and everyone around you that you have the power to become the changes you want to see.

This book describes the program I follow today, the most current evolution of a mental and physical quest that has made me into an internationally recognized race car driver, a *Sports Illustrated* swimsuit model, and the only professional female athlete in the world who competes exclusively against men. It is the program that has changed my life.

It works for me. And it will work for you.

I Gave My Mom Abs!

I know this program will work for you because I've already shared it with hundreds of others—men and women just like you, who lost weight, built muscle, and dramatically changed the way they look and feel.

Pretty Intense is the result of a years-long journey of putting pen to paper—my quest to document the actions I've taken for myself that have delivered the best results, mentally and physically, that I have ever had. Then it was hours and hours of sweating to test and fine-tune every workout so each one is perfect. To top it off, I decided I would cook, style, and photograph all the food myself as I double-checked recipes and created new ones!

In January 2017, I started the *Pretty Intense* Challenge at PrettyIntense.com. More than seven hundred fans signed up to follow the 90-day plan—average men and women just like you who enjoyed the same amazing results I saw, and whose stories appear on these pages.

And as the challenge grew, a community sprouted up. Along with the forums and regular e-mails available on PrettyIntense.com, the PI Tribe (as the team decided to call themselves) even started a Facebook page, *Pretty Intense* People. It was amazing to be able to check in with everyone through social media and see the incredible results they were posting, and, yes, my mom was one of them! I promise you, she is authentically crazy excited about this new way of life, and loves the food and the workouts. At her final weigh-in, she discovered she'd lost eleven pounds in twelve weeks, and she jumped around with joy like a little kid, seriously. Check out my mom! So proud.

Another one of my favorite stories came from Tracey and Shawn Rennecker. Between the two of them, this married couple dropped a total of fifty-two pounds (twenty-one for Shawn, thirty-one for Tracey) in twelve weeks.

But this book isn't about losing weight. It's about changing the shape of your body, and becoming mentally and physically fitter

"Yes, you really can do this!"

BEV PATRICK, 59
Indianapolis, Indiana

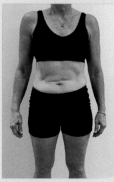
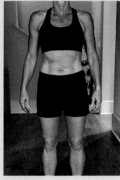

BEFORE   AFTER

Mom was one of the very first people to join the *Pretty Intense* Tribe. And despite her initial fears that she wouldn't be able to keep up, she not only loved the program—she saw amazing results as well.

"Danica was here for the holidays, and she said, 'Mom, you've really got to sign up for this program.' I've worked out for years, but I was never superfit. I was concerned about whether or not I'd be able to keep up with Danica's workouts—I'm not 30 anymore."

But like others who tried the challenge, Mom was surprised by how easy the program was to start and to stick to. "You look at the workouts and see that you're supposed to do burpees and mountain climbers and other things you've never done, and you think, 'Oh I could never do that!' But then you do them and you feel great. It's a gradual growing of confidence that yes, you really can do this. And having week-by-week workouts keeps you accountable; you want to check them all off before the start of the next week."

Pretty Intense hasn't just changed her exercise habits; it's completely changed the way Mom eats, even though she doesn't feel the need to follow the nutrition plan exactly. "I try to just go by Danica's rules for gluten and dairy, and try to eliminate that from my diet," she explains. "And the way I feel is so different—you just don't get that bloated feeling and those highs and lows. And then the weight started coming off. In 12 weeks I lost 11 pounds, and that's a lot for me. And I know I put on muscle, so I must have lost even more fat. I tell people, don't go by the scale, go by how you feel. And I feel so much better."

In fact, the biggest change was a completely unexpected one: "I'm in that beautiful twilight of menopause," says Mom. "After 4 or 5 weeks my hot flashes completely stopped. That was a life changer. I definitely have more energy, and more confidence. Just try it!"

> "If you can set aside thirty minutes a day for yourself, you can manage this program."

LAURA GOODALE, 29
Manteno, Illinois

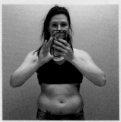
BEFORE

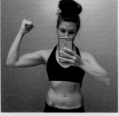
AFTER

As a business project analyst for a large insurance company, Laura is lucky enough to be able to work from home. But she's unlucky enough to be spending nine to ten hours a day sitting in front of a computer screen. "I was active, but I would not consider myself fit," she says.

That changed when she took on the *Pretty Intense* Challenge. She not only lost fourteen pounds and 6 percent of her body fat, but she saw her body shape change dramatically—her stomach flattened and her arms grew leaner and more defined. Her favorite change, though, can't be seen from the outside: "It's my energy levels. I always used to have to take my afternoon nap for an hour, but after starting this program I have no need to nap. I have so much energy!"

She says the biggest difference between *Pretty Intense* and other workout programs she's tried is variety. "The other programs I've tried had the same workouts and the same structure and didn't present variation. The lack of excitement and mystery personally led me to fail. I enjoy not knowing what is coming next; your body responds best to challenge and change."

The biggest advantage Laura found with *Pretty Intense* was its flexibility. "I gave myself two rest days, and if there was a day I was just not able to get that workout in, I had the flexibility to exchange it for a rest day. If you can set aside thirty minutes a day for yourself, you can manage this program."

In addition to newfound energy, Laura has found another new thing to love: breakfast. "I was not a breakfast person before I started this journey, and it's probably the one meal I look forward to each day now. My favorite food would have to be a tie between chia pudding and those fabulous pancakes!"

In the end, what Laura came away with, besides a new body, was a newfound sense of confidence. "I have never felt as confident as I do today. Mentally and physically I put my mind to it and I conquered it. I feel stronger and actually give a damn about myself. This program conditioned me to do the unthinkable."

and stronger in every possible way. That's why you'll measure your results not just with a scale, but with an exclusive fitness test I've created that will tell you just how much stronger and healthier you're becoming—even as your waistline shrinks and your entire body becomes leaner and more defined.

Change Your Body, Change Your Life

That said, this book isn't a fitness book, and it's not a diet book. It's a whole-life plan for building strength, confidence, and happiness inside and out. It's about feeling good about who you are, not just how you look. It's about taking control of your life as well as your body. It's about being as strong, empowered, and, yes, as intense as possible, in every aspect of your life.

Pretty Intense is a three-part plan:

- **A mental-conditioning regimen** to bring peacefulness, mindfulness, and a quiet confidence into your life. I'll give you a series of simple self-tests to help you learn more about yourself and set and achieve goals that will help you redefine your life. (You'll follow along with me as I show you how I use a wide range of life-affirming hobbies and habits to keep me focused and disciplined.) And I'll share some simple, inspiring thoughts and mantras to help you get stronger and more confident in the gym, in the kitchen, and in all your personal relationships.

> "I was wearing large, baggy men's sweatpants and stealing my husband's XL T-shirts, because none of my clothes fit anymore. I was ashamed of myself and how I looked. Now, after completing the Pretty Intense *program*, I've lost over thirty pounds, and I have gone from a size 13 down to a size 8. Thank you for being the amazingly strong woman that you are and for putting together the Pretty Intense *Challenge. You rock."*
>
> **KATHRYN CHALMERS**

- **A high-intensity fitness program** based on the workouts I've created for myself, and incorporating the latest science on improving metabolism, burning fat, timing meals and exercise, and maximizing your effort so every workout counts. (You can even watch me demonstrating these moves for you in a series of easy-to-follow videos you'll find on PrettyIntense.com.)

- **A real-food-based eating plan** that strips away unnecessary carbs and processed foods while showing you the basics of the most important weight-loss skill you'll ever learn: cooking. (I'm including fifty of my favorite recipes.) I'll show you how to follow a delicious and satisfying diet that quickly and effectively shrinks and sculpts your body while giving you *more* energy, not less! In fact, what people rave about the most is how good they feel, and how much energy they have for every aspect of their lives.

> "My energy levels are way up. I don't feel nearly as run-down as I used to. My head feels more clear. My confidence is up. I think my relationships are better with my family, friends, and my husband."
>
> **MELISSA SCHILZ**

You'll begin the same way the *PI* Tribe began: with a fitness test you'll use to discover exactly where your body is at today. And you'll be able to measure after twelve weeks how much fitter and stronger you've become.

We are on a journey, my friends.

A journey to a fitter you.

A journey to a happier you.

A journey to a physically stronger you.

And most important, a journey to a mentally stronger you.

And I am going to be with you the whole way! I promise!

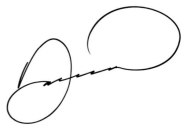

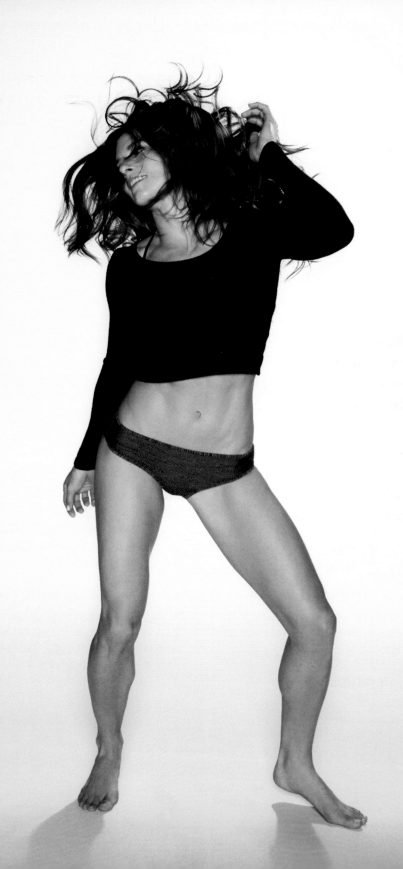

CONTENTS

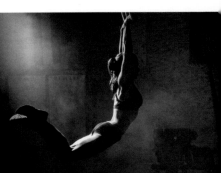

Part One: The *Pretty Intense* Mind

Chapter 1 // Explore Your Mind River

Get in the happiness habit, and learn how to direct your thoughts so you're always thinking, and moving, toward a stronger body and a stronger mind. **page 33**

Chapter 2 // Build Your WOman Cave

Carve out a place that's just for you, and unleash your full potential—emotionally, creatively, and physically. **page 43**

Chapter 3 // Open Up to Nature

Scientists would call it quantum physics, but most of us call it vibes: become attuned to them and discover the power to attract what you want for your life. **page 51**

Chapter 4 // Dream Big

Dare to step out of your comfort zone— physically, emotionally, intellectually. Look for a peak that's dizzyingly high. That's where we're headed! **page 59**

Chapter 5 // Be Your Own BFF

A best friend is someone you can always rely on, someone you can be honest with, someone who will never judge you. Here's how to be that person—for yourself! **page 67**

Part Two: The *Pretty Intense* Body

Part Three: *Pretty Intense* Food

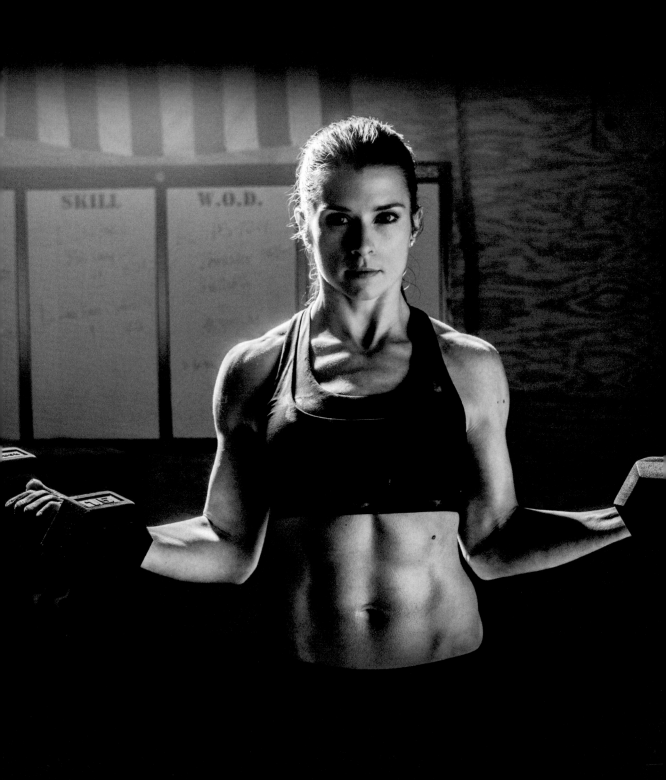

INTRODUCTION

I am not going to bore you with my life story.

This book is about giving you the information and experiences that have brought me to the place I am *now*. But to be clear, between the ages of fourteen and thirty-four, I tried just about every style of eating and exercising known to man.

And at age thirty-four, *Pretty Intense* was born.

Pretty Intense describes more than just my diet and fitness program; it describes the way I approach everything in life. That mind-set has brought me success in so many ways, but it's also brought me some things that are more important: health, happiness, and a deeper appreciation for the simple things in life. And that's what I want to share with you. Yes, the program in this book will boost your metabolism, shrink and tone your body, and give you more energy than you've ever had. But it will give you something even more powerful: the confidence to set new goals—and truly achieve them.

I began developing the *Pretty Intense* plan in early 2016. My job doesn't allow for time off, so as a woman driven to succeed at all costs, I decided to undergo IVF treatment to freeze my eggs. I wanted a backup plan—or maybe someday an actual plan! Friends and doctors said that my body would go back to normal after I had a regular cycle. I was shocked by the weight gain I experienced from the hormone shots. It was the first time I really understood the power of hormones and why it's so difficult for women to lose weight after a pregnancy—or for anyone, man or woman, to drop pounds after a significant hormonal shift. Even though I was eating the same way and took only two weeks off from exercising, my body had changed. I had extra fat on me, and it was not coming off with my normal workouts. I realized that if I was going to

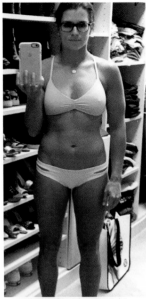

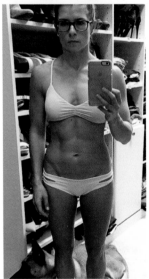

I've been a professional athlete all of my adult life, and I've been training hard since my teens. But even at my level of fitness, the *Pretty Intense* program changed my body more than any program I've ever followed.

look and feel the way I wanted to, I was going to have to do something different.

That "something different" is what you hold in your hands. It's a new way of eating and working out that has given me my best body ever, hormones be damned. And it will do the same for you.

How I Became *Pretty Intense*

One of the earliest lessons I learned in my career was this: the most powerful thing about you is your mind.

That's what makes this book different from any other diet and fitness book on the market. Yes, I'm going to teach you how to eat and exercise to reshape your physique, but first, I'm going to give you the tools you need to bring focus and discipline into your life—tools that are essential to reaching your diet and fitness goals. These are the mental and emotional strategies I use not just when I'm racing at two hundred miles per hour, but when I'm managing and engaging in every aspect of my life, from planting my garden to executing my workout to spending the best possible time with the people I love.

So many of us begin a new fitness or diet plan, or make a promise or a resolution to ourselves, only to drop out after a few weeks or a few months, and that makes sense to me. What makes us think we can change our bodies and our behaviors without changing the way we think about ourselves first?

The fact is, we are all creatures of habit, and the biggest habit of all is our way of thinking. Our lives are the sum of our actions, and our actions come from our thoughts. If we think we're not motivated enough, not smart enough, not good enough, then our actions will reflect those beliefs. If you're in the mental habit of backing down from difficult challenges, of giving up when things get tough, of letting slide commitments that you made to yourself and to others, this mind-set will reflect in your actions, and in the results of your day-in, day-out life.

On the other hand, if you train yourself to habitually push forward when a problem arises, to confront challenges head-on, to stick with difficult situations even when it's not comfortable or convenient, you'll begin to effect change, in body and mind.

> "If you want something you've never had, you have to do something you've never done."
>
> —THOMAS JEFFERSON

Do you feel like you're doing what you were put on Earth to do? Are you excited about the day ahead? Do you come away at the end of the day feeling as though you've made another step toward your goals? *Pretty Intense* will teach you how to get into the right state of mind to do all those things. You'll learn how to confront difficult situations and master them quickly and honestly; how to create a positive energy that will give you confidence in any social or professional situation; and how to fall in love with your own company in a way that brings stillness and calm into your life so that you can truly enjoy the company of others without using them as a means of escape. These are among the tools you need to begin changing your body, and your life. With this newfound confidence, nothing will stop you from getting where you want to go!

That's what *Pretty Intense* has to offer.

Get Strong—from the Inside Out

When was the last time you made a resolution? *I am going to eat healthier. I am going to work out every day. I am going to save more money. I am going to be nicer to people.*

Here's my yearly resolution: *I am not going to make any resolutions.*

Resolutions are nothing more than momentary decisions to effect permanent changes, and they don't work for exactly that reason. If it were so easy to eat right, exercise more, and pursue our dreams, we'd all be doing it every single day, and we'd all be lean, healthy, and happy.

Look around. How's that working out?

To get what we truly want, we need to go deeper.

Pretty Intense will get you out of the resolution/relapse/regret cycle by asking you to do just one thing: the next healthy thing. Together, we'll decide *just for today* to exercise; to make *just this next meal* a healthy one; to tackle *just this one problem* and bring it to resolution. And, over time, brick by brick, we're going to build a new and amazing you.

We'll do it by changing your habits, starting from the inside. (Remember, habits are nothing more than individual actions you take over and over again.) So let's make this easy for ourselves!

Take exercise, for example. I know that there will be days when you wake up full of energy, the sun streaming through your windows, the birds chirping—days when you can't wait to break a sweat and feel fully alive. But there will also be days when the rain is pouring, the kids are screaming, your mind is spinning, and the idea of working out seems like just too much to bear.

I designed the *Pretty Intense* Workouts for *those* days. When it comes to exercise, motivation is job one. That's why you'll begin this program with the *Pretty Intense* Fit Test, a simple workout that will test you physically and mentally. You'll record your time, and you'll revisit the Fit Test again at the end of the program to see real, undeniable proof of how much stronger and healthier you're becoming.

And except for the Fit Test, you'll never do the same workout twice.

Intensity Is the Key to Everything

If anyone has ever told you that you've gained weight because you don't exercise enough, or because you're not motivated enough, or because you're too stressed and too busy, I can almost guarantee they're wrong. In fact, studies show that the average American gets more exercise today than he or she did twenty years ago, while eating about the same number of calories.

The problem isn't time, effort, or motivation. It's intensity. You need to work hard enough to be great.

Too many of us work out all the time without seeing results, because the workouts we're doing simply aren't effective at boosting our metabolism. Burning calories on the stair climber or running on the treadmill will shrink you a little, but it won't help you reshape your body. It won't give you a flat belly, sleek thighs, strong arms, and a tight, firm butt.

The *Pretty Intense* Workout will. It brings intensity back into your life, resetting your metabolism with brief, high-energy workouts that will program your body to burn the maximum amount of fat—not just when you're working out, but all day long. As you reset your internal calorie furnace with a combination of body-weight exercises, resistance training, and aerobic conditioning, you'll begin to see results on an almost daily basis.

Pretty Intense is based on a simple philosophy: it all comes down to intensity. That's true in every aspect of life, but especially in the exercise arena. This workout plan will get you in and out fast—without the need for a gym, expensive equipment, or rearranging your already complex life.

> "Everything you want is on the other side of fear."
>
> —JACK CANFIELD

High-intensity interval training, or HIIT, is the style of workout we'll be focusing on. HIIT refers simply to a workout in which you go hard, at maximum intensity, for a certain amount of time, then back off for a "recovery" period before going at it hard again. I'll show you a combination of fitness plans that includes weights and cardio, with plenty of short workouts (and the occasional longer one), and I'll keep you motivated and challenged. Plus, like me, you'll utilize a series of inspirational phrases (use mine or develop your own with my Magic Mantra Maker) to keep you moving forward—literally.

And throughout, I'll show you exactly what works for me, while introducing you to some of the newest science that informs my approach to fitness, food, and life.

Feed Your Body, Feed Your Soul

I have been a student of nutrition since I was fourteen, and I've experimented with every diet trend that's come along in the last two decades: I've eaten low-fat. I've eaten low-carb. I've made everything whole wheat. I've done dairy-free, gluten-free—you name it,

I've tried it and tweaked it to fit my lifestyle. But the biggest lesson I've learned about diet is this: you need to eat more simply, and in order to do that, you need to have control, and you need to not be afraid of your own kitchen.

In fact, if there is one piece of health and fitness advice I would give to anyone, it is this: learn how to cook.

The way we eat today—even food commonly accepted as "healthy," from brown rice cakes to baked potato chips—has the effect of basically slowing our metabolism, undermining our body's own internal fat-burning systems. Once you learn how food is really prepared, you'll begin to understand why the food at your favorite chain restaurant tastes different: the baked salmon (it's covered with butter!), the pasta sauce (it's loaded with sugar!), even the "grilled" chicken (it's actually fried with vegetable oil!). You'll understand what all those seventeen-syllable words on food labels mean, and why you should avoid them. And you'll finally gain control of your food, your diet, and your life.

More important, you'll never feel hungry. In fact, you'll find yourself eating more food—and more delicious food—than ever before.

The *Pretty Intense* Diet is a Paleo-friendly program featuring dozens of delicious recipes I've built using simple dietary principles that form the basis of my personal nutrition plan: eat real food! It's not about bland, boring rice and beans; on this plan, I'll show you how to grill the perfect steak, caramelize onions to dress an amazing hamburger, and turn even vegetables into savory and irresistible stars of any meal, all the while stripping away the unnecessary and unhealthy additives that can cause weight gain.

And these foods and recipes are just the beginning. I believe the key to becoming a success in the kitchen is to unleash one's own creativity. I'll guide you through the processes I use to create my own recipes so you can enjoy the same great foods I eat every day while developing your own repertoire of delicious go-tos.

So what do you think?

Can you do this?

I know you can. And I'm going to be with you every step of the way.

The *Pretty Intense* Program at a Glance

Nutrition

The idea for this eating plan is to focus on eating REAL food! Meat, fish, vegetables, fruit, nuts, seeds, and healthy fats. I want you to eat foods as close to their original form as you can. Look at the ingredients list: in most cases there shouldn't be more than five ingredients, and you should be able to pronounce them all!

Everything you eat should be adding to your well-being, not reducing it. It will be a little tricky for a week or two adjusting your meals and figuring out what foods and combinations you like, but stick it out. I promise, it will be worth it. I can't wait for you to discover new and delicious *simple* foods!

Number of Meals

Three per day—no skipping breakfast!

Number of Snacks

Two or three per day (hunger is your enemy!)

Eat More

Meats, fish, vegetables, fruit, nuts, seeds, coconut oil, olive oil, ghee, avocado oil, nut milks, coconut milk, potatoes, and eggs

Avoid

Dairy (including milk, cheese, and yogurt), wheat flour–based foods (including whole-grain and white bread, pasta, and pastries), soy, sugar, and artificial sweeteners

Cut Down On

Legumes (peas, beans, lentils, and peanuts) and grains (corn, oats, rice, quinoa)

Calories

Don't sweat it! Eat the right foods at the right times, and the calories will take care of themselves.

Cheat Days and Cheat Meals

Since there are occasions when we have very little control over what we fuel our bodies with, I don't plan cheat meals. That way, when I don't eat quite as well, it's no big deal. Do your very best all the time, and you will stay ahead! Cheat meals are a gimmick that a lot of diet marketers use to make their plans more palatable. It's not something you need. Yes, there will be special occasions when you will indulge, and that's okay! No need to feel guilty when celebrating, finally getting to relax, or eating something you rarely get! Just get back to eating your *Pretty Intense* diet at your next meal! What you'll discover is that you'll no longer crave unhealthy food, because of how good you feel. If you don't yet believe me, you will. (Imagine a life in which you don't even want bad food!)

Alcohol

It's allowed, but remember that each time you indulge, you'll reduce your results. When you do drink, avoid beer, and cocktails made with sugary mixers. (Those frozen margaritas and piña coladas are the worst!) Instead, choose wine, or cocktails made with clear liquor and club soda with lemon slices (not tonic water, which has lots of added sugar).

Hunger Is Your Enemy

The first thing you might notice when you see this nutrition plan is, there's a lot of food! In fact, you'll probably be eating much more often on this plan than you're used to. How can that possibly translate to weight loss?

Because the right food, eaten at the right time, is the most effective weight-loss tool out there. More than exercise, much more than "dieting" or calorie restriction, fueling your body with healthy, high-protein, high-fiber, nutrient-dense food at regular intervals throughout the day will have the greatest impact on the shape and size of your body.

Eating the *Pretty Intense* Way

To help your body start burning fat and give you the energy you need, you'll focus on a series of super-healthy food groups, each of which spark metabolism in its own particular way, while giving your overall health a boost. Here's a general idea of the foods you'll enjoy on this program:

Breakfast

- 2 eggs; ½ sweet potato, shredded and sautéed into hash; and ½ avocado
- Ground bison with ½ roasted acorn squash, ½ diced apple, and ½ avocado
- Ground beef (85% lean or leaner) with sautéed spinach and sautéed diced butternut squash

- Chia pudding with berries, gluten- and grain-free granola, coconut flakes, and a drizzle of honey (to make a batch of chia seed pudding, combine 1 can light coconut milk or ½ cup almond milk and ½ cup chia seeds, stir, and let it sit in the fridge for 20 minutes, or overnight)

Lunch

- Grilled chicken, mixed greens, avocado
- Loaded veggie salad with salmon

- Sweet potato and salmon
- Bunless burger and a salad

Dinner

- Rotisserie chicken, roasted Brussels sprouts, and carrots
- Spiral zucchini "pasta" with olive oil and tomatoes, grilled chicken or ground beef, and a side salad

- Grass-fed beef or bison steak with grilled bell peppers and zucchini
- Roasted squash and sweet potatoes will be your best friends to bulk up your meals

Snacks

- Apple with nut butter
- ½ banana with a handful of almonds
- ½ avocado with a squeeze of lime and sprinkling of salt

- Protein shake with a nut milk, frozen ½ banana and 1 cup strawberries, almond butter, hemp seeds, and chia seeds
- Healthy fats like nuts, nut butters, avocados, and animal fats will keep you full

Desserts

- 72% or more dark chocolate (make sure it has greater than 72% cacao and says so on the label—it is packed with filling fiber and healthy antioxidants)

- Chocolate chia pudding with coconut flakes, cocoa nibs, and a drizzle of maple syrup
- Mixed berries

Fitness

For the past year, I've been working hard in the gym, adapting my own exercise regimen into a plan that's perfectly suited for anyone. This 12-week program starts off moderately challenging and ramps up from there. Each week will include:

- 3—interval cardio sessions
- 1—upper body workout
- 1—lower body workout
- 1—abs workout
- 1—long circuit

Each workout is designed to take between 20 and 25 minutes, except for the "long circuit," which will take between 30 and 45 minutes.

Equipment needed

- Chair/bench
- Jump rope
- Slam ball
- Mat
- Tabata timer. I personally use the MyWOD app, but there are lots of apps out there.
- Set of dumbbells (10 pounds)
- Optional—additional dumbbells (5 and 15 pounds)

Only you know your schedule and lifestyle, so I can't impose my regimen on you. But if I were to recommend when to do these workouts, and in what order, it would look like this:

MON	TUES	WED	THURS	FRI	SAT	SUN
cardio (A.M.) upper body (P.M.)	lower body (A.M. OR P.M.)	cardio (A.M.) abs (P.M.)	cardio (A.M. OR P.M.)	off	long circuit (A.M. OR P.M.)	off

This is just how I would do it, and following this regimen would provide me with maximum strength to perform each workout to the highest of my ability.

You'll notice that on a couple of days, I'm recommending two workouts in one day. I would like you to get comfortable with that idea, even if you just want to stick with one workout a day in the beginning, or to stack two workouts together to save time. But my hope is that at some point you will be able to work out twice a day on occasion, which will really stoke your metabolism and change it up on your body.

Over the course of the next 12 weeks you'll never do the same workout more than once. There are two reasons why: First, it's a lot more fun if the exercises, structure, and rep schemes change. Dah! And second, I want to keep your body *and* your mind constantly challenged and tested. You will not only become stronger physically, but mentally. You will no longer be afraid when you see a hundred reps of something in a workout, because you've done it! And it wasn't really that bad. It also teaches you that when you have only ten reps to do, it's going to seem really easy!

"I lost my love handles."

**MICHAEL TASCONA, 37
Tampa, Florida**

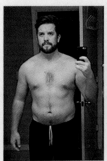 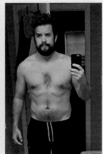

BEFORE   AFTER

A former lineman working on high cable towers—sometimes rappelling down to them from a helicopter—Michael had always been physically active. But a few years ago he moved to Florida to start a new career in sales. "That's a different ballgame," he says. "It's not physical at all—it's all eating and drinking."

Despite running, taking some exercise classes, and following diet advice from his sister, a nutritionist, Michael was starting to see his weight creep up. Soon, he was up to 207 pounds, and with his travel schedule, working out more just wasn't an option. He needed to work out smarter. Then he found *Pretty Intense*.

"My friends were following Danica on Instagram and I saw her post about this program. When I first did the Fit Test I thought, Wow, this is going to be intense. But the first workouts weren't intimidating at all."

It didn't take long for that extra business-meal weight to start to fall away. "I lost my love handles, and that was a big thing. My goal was to get down below 200, but I lost 14 pounds, and I'm down to 193." Michael admits he's got a love/hate relationship with some of the exercises: "Abs day sucks, but it's also one of my favorite workouts." And now that his love handles have melted away, he can start to see the result of his efforts.

If there's one overriding idea with this program, it's this: I want you to crank up the intensity, at least for a short amount of time. This isn't "slow and steady," and it isn't "lift and then rest." You should be working a lot more than resting!

That said, if something hurts, then stop or modify the exercise! You should modify especially if you're feeling pain in joints like your knees, hips, elbows, or shoulders. You might also have to modify the workout if running outside isn't possible due to weather, like a snowstorm or freezing temperatures in Chicago in January—*brrrr*! Here are some options to replace running in the cardio workouts (the following moves are written in my preferred order of effectiveness to get your heart rate up): jump rope, stair taps, skipping, high knees, jumping jacks, butt kickers, or running stairs (if you have a lot of them, such as in a high rise). Also, if you have a rowing machine or bike, they would work as well.

But don't confuse "it hurts" with "it's too hard." That's merely a mental hurdle. It's not any harder to keep going slowly than it is to stop and then have to talk yourself into starting again. My trick when I have to take a break is to count to three or five and then start again.

These workouts will be over before you know it, so work hard! I'm sure the time you have to work out is limited; don't waste it resting. Give it your best effort for the short amount of time you have to not only look better but *feel* better, too!

Before We Start . . .
The *Pretty Intense* Fit Test

Well, let's get started! I have created a fitness test for you to complete beforehand and then again at the end of the program. This will help you recognize how far you will have come over the next 12 weeks from a performance standpoint. Remember to record your time, and you'll marvel at how dramatically it drops. Good luck!

For easy-to-follow videos of me doing these exercises (and all the exercises you'll find in this book), go to PrettyIntense.com.

FIT TEST—for time:

- 100 air squats
- 100 knee push-ups
- 100 butterfly sit-ups
- 100 lunges (50 each side)

NOTE: Most people will need between 30 and 60 minutes to complete this test. As you get fitter, your time will quickly drop below half an hour. Most of the folks who completed the program got their times down below 20 minutes total.

Me? My best time is 9:01.

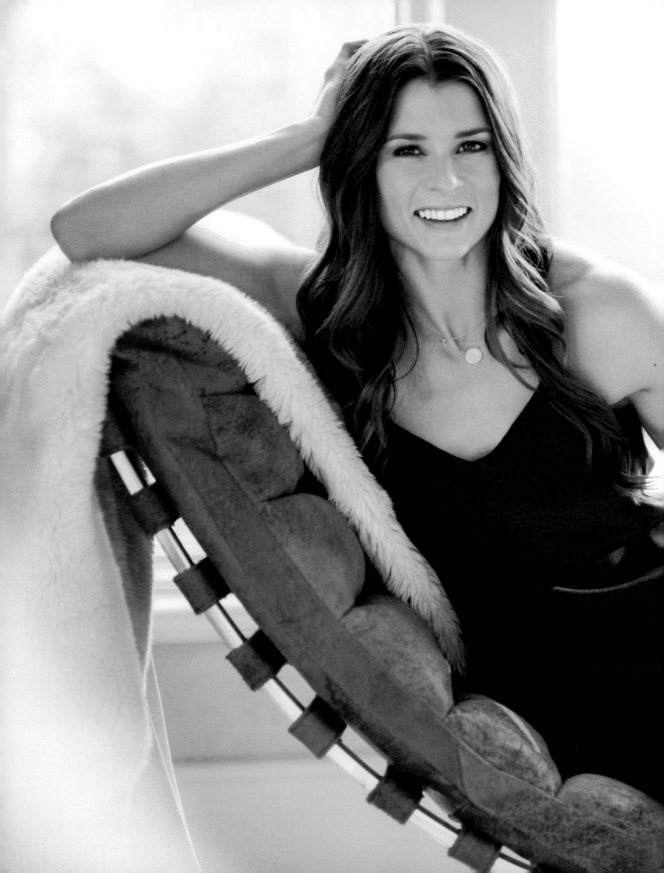

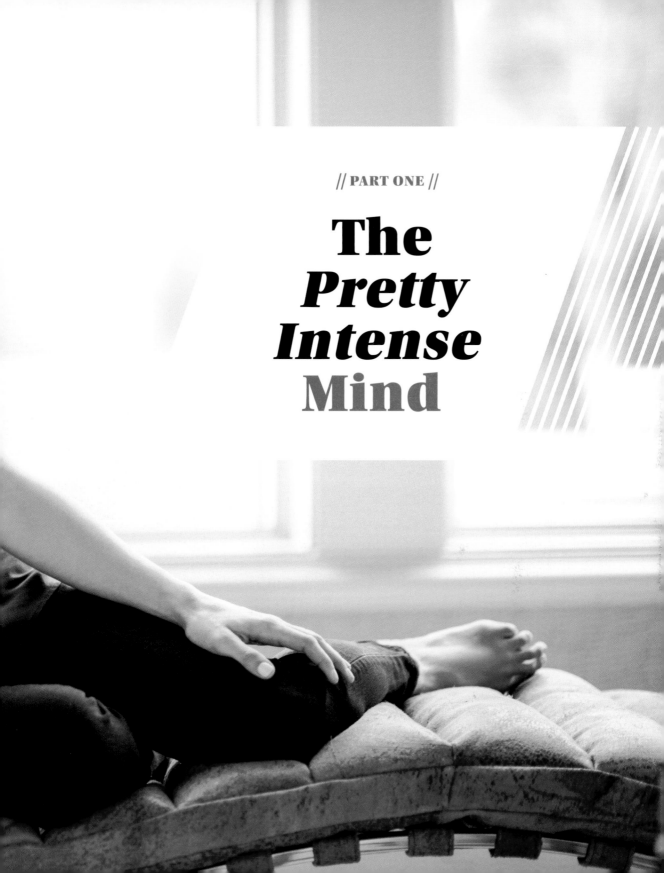

// PART ONE //

The *Pretty Intense* Mind

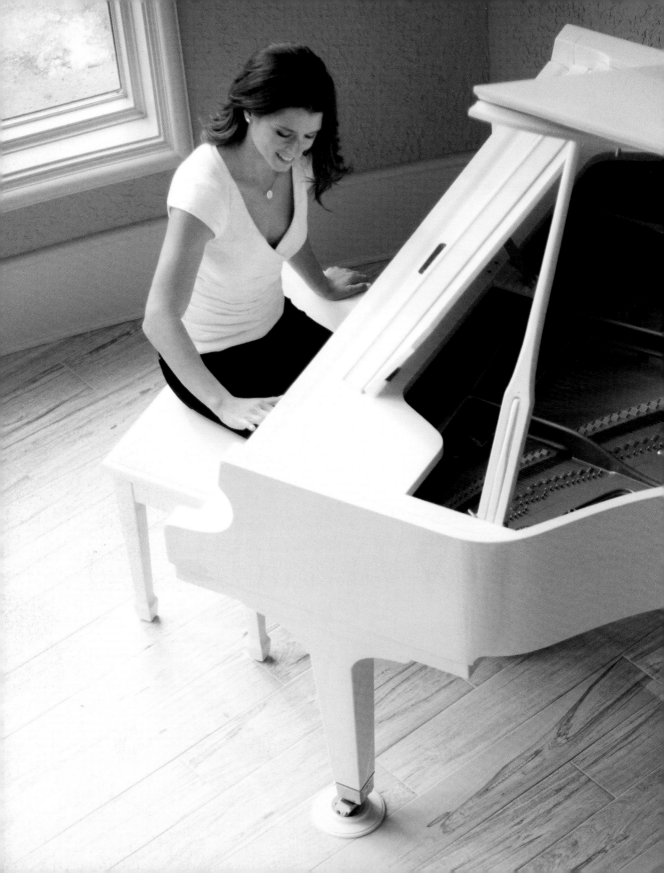

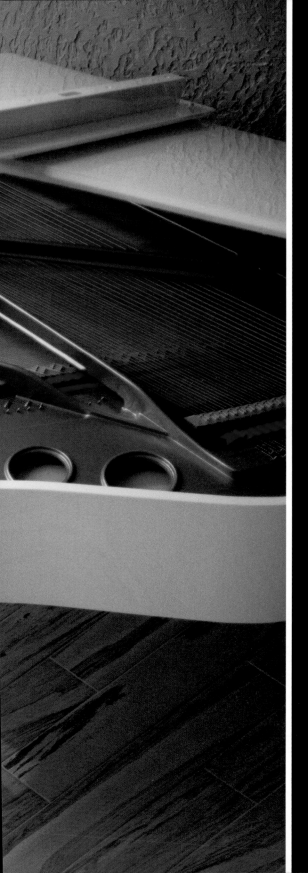

CHAPTER 1

EXPLORE YOUR MIND RIVER

I have discovered the secret to spiritual peace and total happiness, and I'm going to reveal it in this chapter.

You might be thinking right now, "Spiritual peace and total happiness are nice and all, but what about the abs? Can I just get the abs?"

Well, yes, you can, but it's going to be a lot harder if you don't get your mind right.

I try like hell to be happy every day—happy on my own terms, without needing anybody else's praise or affections. Being happy is like being fit: it takes work; it takes exercise. When I stop working on my personal happiness, I start to let in feelings that lead to unhealthy choices—being unkind to people, not prioritizing my own well-being—and sometimes I start to lose who I really am deep down. Being unhappy is a sign that I'm not working hard enough.

Happiness is, after all, a state of mind, and the only person who has the ability to change your mind—the only person who can make you happy—is you. In Eastern philosophy, it's called "living your dharma"—the feeling of contentment that comes with knowing that you are doing what you were put on Earth to do. That's what this chapter is designed to help you achieve through attracting the kinds of energies that will bring you closer to your higher self instead of your ego.

Understand Your "Mind River"

When I'm racing, I can't afford to think about all the terrible things that could happen to me, or what I *don't* want to be doing. I have to focus on what I *do* want! A vehicle naturally follows its driver's eyes, and glancing at the dangers ahead or alongside me is a sure way of driving right into them. A driver must always look at the openings, not the obstacles.

The same is true in life. If your thoughts are always pointing toward the negative—if you're repeatedly pondering your own shortcomings, dwelling on your failures, or seeing the obstacles up ahead of you—you will inevitably crash right into them.

> "It isn't what you have, or who you are, or where you are, or what you are doing that makes you happy or unhappy. It is what you think about."
>
> —DALE CARNEGIE

I like to think of it this way: Our thoughts are like a river flowing over rock. Over time, the water wears a path into the rock, a path that becomes more and more permanent the deeper it's cut. When we think negative thoughts about ourselves or others, we're cutting a path that eventually will become if not permanent, then at least harder and harder to escape. They call it a rut for just that reason: we get a wheel stuck in that negative space and just keep digging it deeper.

Thoughts are powerful things. Over time, your thoughts become your words. Your words become your actions. And your actions become your character.

You know that person in your life—and if you're lucky, you have more than one—who always seems to make you feel good when you're around them? That person who oozes joy in a way that cuts through whatever bad mood you're in? Why are they like that?

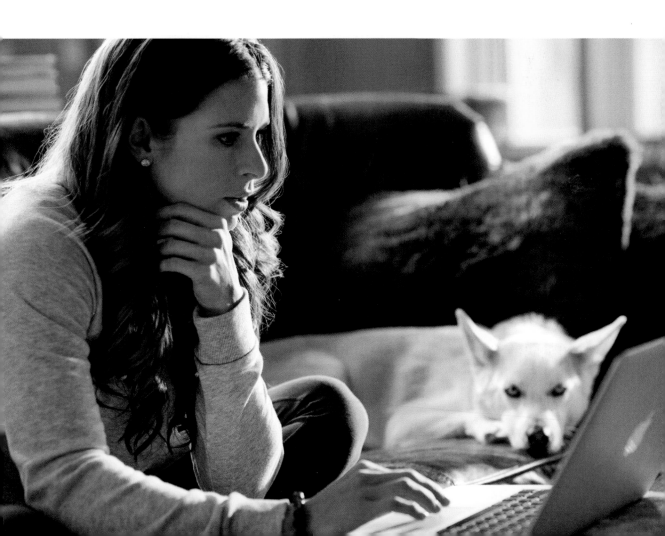

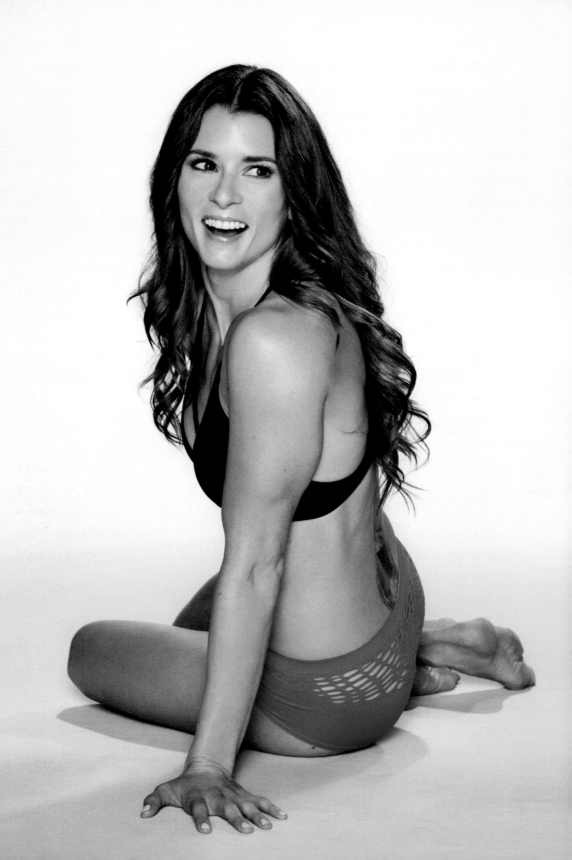

They're like that because they think in a positive manner—their mind river cuts a path of hope and happiness, and each day they let that path grow a little deeper.

For some of us, this comes naturally, but for most of us, it's a habit that needs to be learned and practiced. And if that's the kind of person you want to be—the kind who attracts others through pure positivity, the kind who's always happy—then it starts with a conscious effort to change the way you think.

It starts with your mind river.

> "Happiness is when what you think, what you say, and what you do are in harmony."
>
> —MAHATMA GANDHI

Three Rules of Happiness

I'm not going to lie and tell you it's easy. Like I said, I try like hell to be a happy person every day, but it's tough. It comes with a lot of practice, and it comes from creating rules for myself, rules that inspire me to be better every day.

RULE #1: Flow in the right direction.

Remember, your thoughts are extremely powerful. We are creatures of habit—I know I am, for sure, and I work every day to promote good habits (eating right, going to the gym, meditating, calling friends and family) and avoid the bad ones. That includes habits of the mind; I don't want to be thinking negatively about myself or others, or letting resentments, jealousies, and insecurities get hold inside of me. Positive thinking is a habit; practice it, and it will start to become natural.

Be light. Be positive. Keep your mind river flowing in the right direction.

RULE #2: Start by assuming the best.

I try to see the good in people and move through my day with the expectation that pretty much everyone is doing their very best. Sometimes, no matter how positive you may be, you'll get blowback. But we all have moments when our best isn't very good at all. Maybe the person you're having a tough time with has a lot of really awful stuff going on in their life, or they were given some terrible news, and they can't help those dark clouds from rolling out. I'll talk a bit about how to confront negative energy in a later chapter, but right now, let's start with what you can control.

RULE #3: Do the next healthy thing.

You don't have to master these skills all at once. You don't have to completely change your outlook on life in an instant. Just do *the next healthy thing*. With the next decision you make when you close this chapter, make the choice that moves you toward your dream. Then, when you're faced with the next decision after that, do the same thing.

That's all you need to do. Take it one decision at a time.

That's why I hate the idea of "resolutions." When we make a resolution, we try to plan out the next month or the next year. It's a total trap. We can't control what's going to happen down the road; pledging to go to the gym four days a week or to never eat chocolate cake for a year is just a recipe for failure. So forget the future; just make the next healthy choice for yourself right now. When you choose to follow these approaches, you'll find they become easier as time goes on.

Fake It Until You Make It

Look, I am just like everyone else when it comes to having bad days! They happen—it's called life. *But* how I choose to deal with them is a choice. My choice.

If I'm just not feeling it that day, I fake it, like . . . obnoxiously. This was a method I developed early in my Indy car days, when I needed a boost to get over all the haters and days that just made me feel less happy and confident than I wanted to be. I called it my "kittens and rainbows" attitude.

Today, I still rely on the same approach: Whenever I'm filled with self-doubt or I'm not looking forward to the tough day ahead, I tell myself that I'm brimming with con- fidence (thought), I project it out to the world (words), I carry myself like I'm fearless (actions), and in no time, it becomes true (character). Today it comes automatically, but it's not a God-given quality; it took a lot of make-believe for me to master being a happy person in real life. The same goes for my fitness: When I don't want to go to the gym, I put on my coolest gym outfit and just pretend that I'm super-psyched to be there. And guess what? By the time I break a sweat, I'm happy to be exercising again.

Afraid? Fake fearlessness, and you'll be surprised how brave you quickly become.

Unmotivated? Pretend you're a total killer, and in time you'll evolve into one.

Unhappy? Focus on making others happier and more comfortable, and eventually you'll forget you even know how to frown.

> "I now embrace myself for who I am and walk with my head held high."

PATTY BRETZ, 45
Sherrills Ford, North Carolina

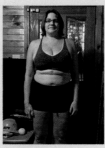 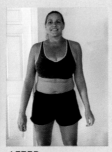

BEFORE   AFTER

An office and procurement manager for a small business, Patty was frustrated by the many exercise programs she'd tried. "P90X, 21-Day Fix, Winsor Pilates—you name it, I've tried it! But I wasn't very disciplined and became frustrated with the results." *Pretty Intense* was a different story altogether. "The biggest difference to me was that the workouts varied and were never the same week after week like other programs." And by week twelve, Patty had shed twenty-five pounds, and five inches from her waist.

And the food! That was a huge part of Patty's success. "I was always a sugar girl and a diet-soda freak," she says. But embracing healthy foods came surprisingly easy on this program. "I was one of those 'yuck' or 'ewww' types before I ever tried something new. But on this plan I fell in love with asparagus, squash, and zucchini. I have even found myself liking sweet potatoes, which were another 'I'm not going to try that!' vegetable."

Now she's not only more confident in the kitchen but in life as well. "I went through a tough time with a divorce and became very self-conscious, as I was told that I didn't look the same as I did when I played volleyball in college. After that, I took the unhealthy route of working out seven days a week while only eating one small meal a day." *Pretty Intense* has not only given her a new body, it's given her a new attitude: "I used to look at workout programs as just a physical aspect of life, but now I view *PI* as a healthy, life-changing journey."

Get in the Happiness Habit

Cultivate good habits. Make it a habit to spot a problem and confront it right then and there. Make it a habit to help others, to put their needs and feelings before your own. Make it a habit to shrug away negative thoughts and let go when you find you're comparing yourself to other people. These habits lead to happiness in the long term.

But the shortest path to happiness—and I truly believe this—is to simply fake being happy. Seriously. There are plenty of times when I feel cranky, but when I do I just "pretend" to be in a good mood by putting a smile on my face, putting my dark thoughts on hold, and being extra nice to others. Inevitably, my self-focus and negativity go away. If I act happy, positive, and confident, sure enough, in no time at all that's actually how I feel, and then I'm ready for anything.

So the first step in being happy? Be happy. The rest of it (yes, even the abs) will follow.

> "The thought manifests as the word;
> the word manifests as the deed;
> the deed develops into habit;
> and habit hardens into character.
> So watch the thought and its
> ways with care, and let it spring
> from love born out of concern
> for all beings."
>
> —GUATAMA BUDDHA

Throughout this book, you'll find a series of quizzes and worksheets that will help you assess where you are in mind, body, and spirit. I suggest you use a pencil (not a pen) for each of the quizzes, because I'm hoping you'll find yourself going back and changing the answers as you progress.

Worksheet: Mind River

I am happiest when I

_____.

My favorite physical feature about myself is

_____.

My favorite thing to do when I have free time is

_____.

If I were to go on vacation anywhere I wanted, it would be to

_____.

If someone were to describe me with one word, it would be

_____.

If I close my eyes and think of my favorite person it would be

_____.

Given one hour of free time, I would

_____.

If someone gave me a million dollars, I would

_____.

The most important thing to me is

_____.

If I could do any job, it would be

_____.

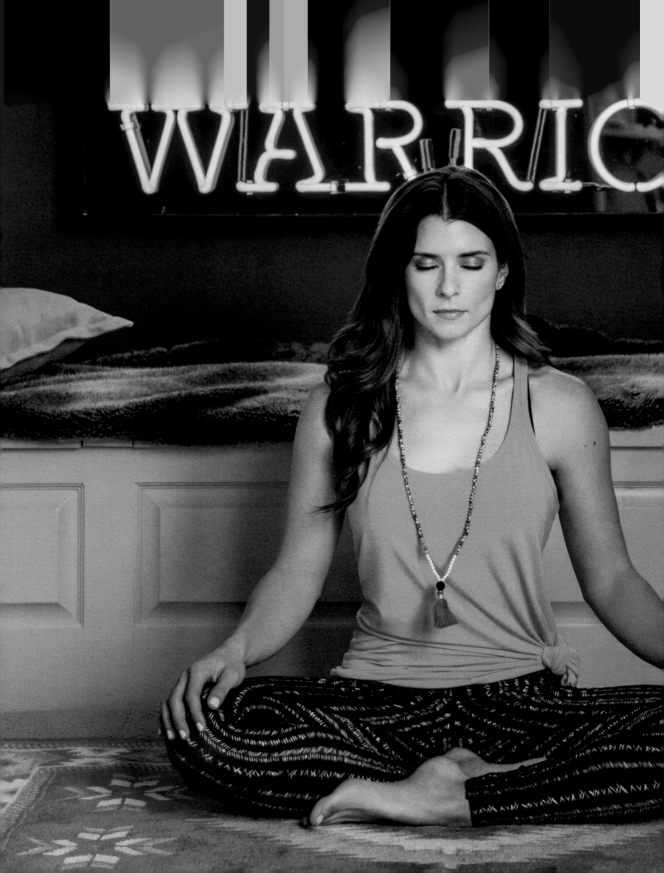

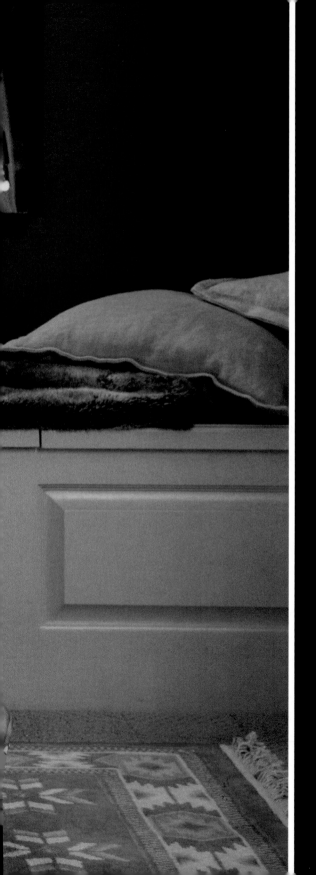

CHAPTER 2

BUILD YOUR WOMAN CAVE

I spend most of my time with my boyfriend, Ricky, and my two dogs, Ella and Dallas, on a converted horse farm outside of Charlotte, North Carolina. We're a small family, but we're a family nonetheless, and as with any family, no matter how big a house we may have, sometimes . . . I need a little space. That's why, a few years ago, I created a small room dedicated just to me. It might have been the smartest thing I ever did.

It started simply because I needed a place to practice yoga and store my art materials, but it evolved into a sacred space. I call it my WOman cave. I happened to choose dark blue as the paint color—which is interesting to me, because in yoga, blue corresponds to the fifth chakra, located in the throat area; energy flowing through this chakra is responsible for helping us speak our truth. I didn't know all that then, but I do now, and I've come to believe that there is no such thing as a coincidence. My WOman cave is where I speak my truth: I filled it with pictures, paintings, and my own creative decorating. I also hung up some of my favorite phrases and motivating mantras (you'll read more about these in an upcoming chapter).

Now I understand why guys started creating man caves. Living with other people is all about making compromises, but a cave of your own can be filled only with things that make *you* happy.

Get Back to Yourself

When I'm not with my family or behind the wheel of a race car, I'm usually doing a photo shoot or an interview, in post-race meetings at the race shop, managing my other businesses, doing conference calls, or traveling for appearances.

But you don't have to be a celebrity to feel those same pressures. Most of us feel the need to be constantly "on"—to present a public face that represents how we want others to perceive us. Even when we're with our loved ones, we're still playing roles—the helpful friend, the doting partner, the firm-but-fair parent.

That's why having a space to call our own is so important. It's an opportunity to forget about other people for a little while: to focus our minds, to clear out the clutter, and to reengage with our passions. In my cave I daydream, I plot and scheme, I sit back and reassess my day and where I am in my life. My personal space is sacred because it's where I discover more about who I am and what I want in life. Taking time to explore these things makes me a better friend, partner, sister, daughter.

It's surprising how little time most of us dedicate to this simple task.

Do I really need a quiet space for this? Can't I do my dreaming and scheming in the gym? Not really, no. Remember, working out is about more than physical intensity; it's about mental intensity as well. When I'm exercising, I'm focusing on my workout; I don't have time for daydreaming and thinking about other things. Spacing out during exercise is a great way to make sure your workout doesn't work.

Make It All About You

I'm lucky enough to have a whole room to myself, but this might not be possible for everyone. It's fine if your "cave" is nothing more than a corner of a room somewhere—a section, wall, table, garage space, *something* that is just for you.

Once you've carved out your spot, fill that space with things you love—especially stuff you've created yourself. Start taking more pictures, frame them, and put them out to see. Any arts, crafts, or projects that you have, put them in one place. Add a little furniture—a table or a chair that you love and think is cool or comfortable. There should be a spot where you can sit, work, lie, meditate, or pray. No one else needs to like the things you put in this space; they are for *you*!

My cave is first and foremost a place to put any little item that makes me happy. I also play whatever music I want in there. The space started simple, as did hobbies like writing and painting, but those hobbies grew, because I had a place for them to grow!

And that's key: you're creating a place where you, and the things you love, can realize their full potential. You will be amazed by what can happen when you send intentions or ideas out into the world. They can manifest into amazing things! That's why they're called "passion projects"!

Exercise Your Gratitude Muscles

People always say they "need a little *me* time," but most of us not only forget to take it, we're *afraid* to take it. A few years ago, researchers conducted a series of eleven studies

> "When I started counting my blessings, my whole life turned around."
>
> **—WILLIE NELSON**

in which they put people in an empty room with nothing but their own thoughts. They reported that "participants typically did not enjoy spending 6 to 15 minutes in a room by themselves with nothing to do but think. . . . [M]any preferred to administer electric shocks to themselves instead of being left alone with their thoughts."

Ouch!

Most of us prefer to be doing something, even if it's unpleasant, to doing nothing at all. Problem is, when we're constantly distracting ourselves, we're numbing ourselves to feelings of real joy. I feel as though my appreciation for everything in my life, good and bad, has become deeper thanks to the time I spend on my own.

I'm able to experience happiness and to appreciate all the things that make life worth living more deeply, because that alone time helps me get in touch with my own feelings. I exercise my gratitude muscles, and it's a workout that works.

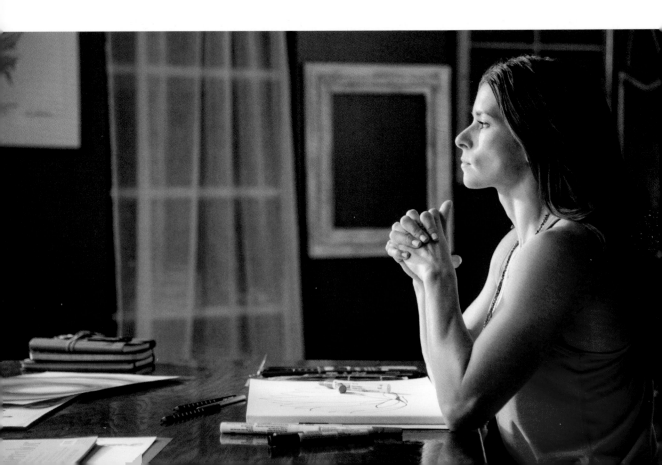

Do Just One Thing

In my WOman cave, I meditate. I paint. I do yoga. I pray. I write. Sometimes I literally do nothing but catch my breath. But no matter what I'm doing, I'm fully engaged in just that one thing. My WOman cave is a multitasking-free zone.

That may not sound exactly revolutionary, but to a certain extent, it is: we're so trained to multitask nowadays that we need laws to prevent us from texting while driving.

And that need to be constantly multitasking has made it harder and harder for us to just be alone with ourselves. Like those test subjects who would rather feel shocks than be still, we can't stand the panicky feeling that time is passing without us "making the most of it"—that we're wasting time and not getting things done.

Researchers say that the average person spends 47 percent of his or her time think-ing about something other than what he or she is doing at the moment. In fact, we're thinking about something else:

- 65 percent of the time when we're taking a shower or brushing our teeth
- 50 percent of the time we're at work
- 40 percent of the time we're exercising
- At least 30 percent of the time we're doing anything else, except . . .
- 10 percent of the time we're having sex

You don't have to spend your alone time doing nothing, but the more you can learn to be alone with yourself—and not needing to constantly distract yourself—the better you'll be able to focus on tasks. I usually shut off my phone, or leave it outside, when I go into my WOman cave. Talking to someone else on the phone isn't "me" time—it's "them" time.

Make sure there's space in your cave to lie down and stretch, meditate, or just be still. The phrase I use is "I give myself permission" to do whatever it is I need to do that makes me feel good. It might be putting off doing dishes, or not calling someone back right away, or warming up dinner instead of making a fresh meal. Teach yourself to be still; it's what we need to recharge our brains and prepare for the challenges we're setting for ourselves. Being quiet, still, and alone helps improve memory and concentration, and it helps us make better decisions. It helps us to feel our own emotions more deeply. The truth lies in the silence. Call it the "gut" or "instinct" or "intuition." Call it what-ever you want. I call it my soul or holy spirit trying to talk to me.

You can still be *Pretty Intense* even when you're doing nothing at all.

The Personal Space Quiz

1 / When I'm not working on something, I feel . . .

    a. At peace.

    b. Worried that I'm not being productive.

    c. Bored and/or anxious.

2 / While reading this chapter, I . . .

    a. Read it all the way through without stopping.

    b. Found my thoughts drifting off and had to force myself back to the page.

    c. Put the book down once or twice and got involved with something else.

3 / When I'm alone, I feel . . .

    a. Happy.

    b. Like other people are having more fun than me.

    c. Restless and discontent.

4 / When I want to work on something, I . . .

    a. Just get started.

    b. Wait for a moment when I can catch my breath, then dive in.

    c. Put it off until the right time, which never seems to come.

5 / If I have to stop something midway through, I often . . .

    a. Pick it right back up when the time is right.

    b. Can't find where I put the items I need the next day.

    c. Can't seem to get back to the task no matter what.

6 / My mind most often feels . . .

    a. Organized and focused.

    b. Like I'm struggling to find balance.

    c. Chaotic and under siege.

7 / If I'm home alone for the night, I will definitely . . .

  a. Find a creative way to use my time.

  b. Watch TV or surf the web.

  c. Panic.

8 / The last time I turned off my phone was . . .

  a. Within the last twenty-four hours.

  b. Sometime in the last week or two.

  c. There's an off switch?

9 / Compared to other people, my life is . . .

  a. Unique and not really comparable.

  b. Better than others' most of the time.

  c. Not up to par most of the time.

10 / Where are my keys?

  a. Right where they belong.

  b. Probably in one of two places.

  c. I have no idea, as usual.

HOW YOU SCORED: This test measures two things: stillness and your gratitude. The more A's you circled, the better you are at calming your mind and counting your blessings. B's indicate you're probably making a conscious effort to capture grace and gratitude, but you're often still busy keeping up with the Joneses, if not the Kardashians. C, in this case, stands for chaos; finding a place for yourself and spending more time in quiet meditation could really help.

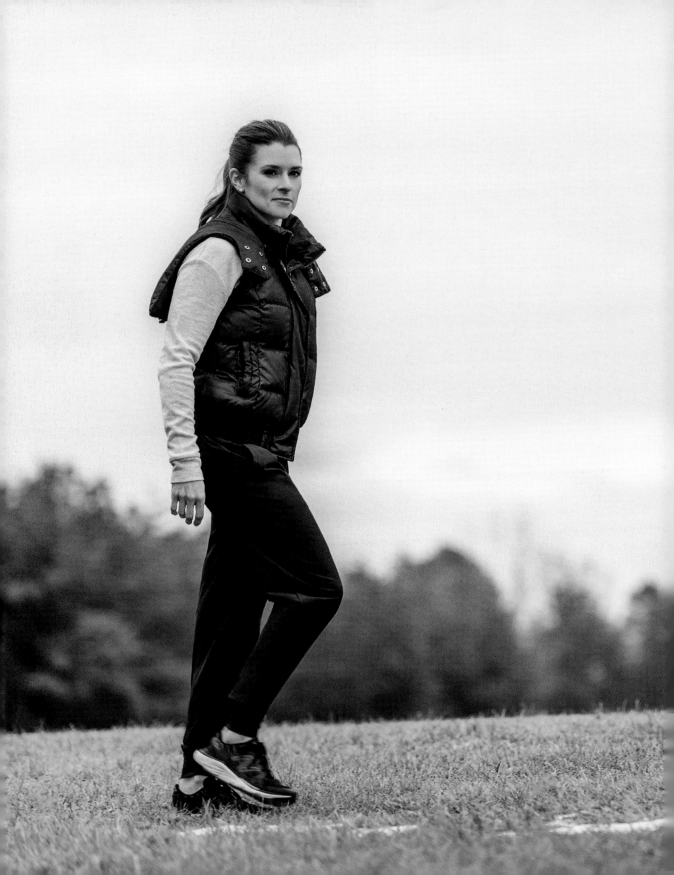

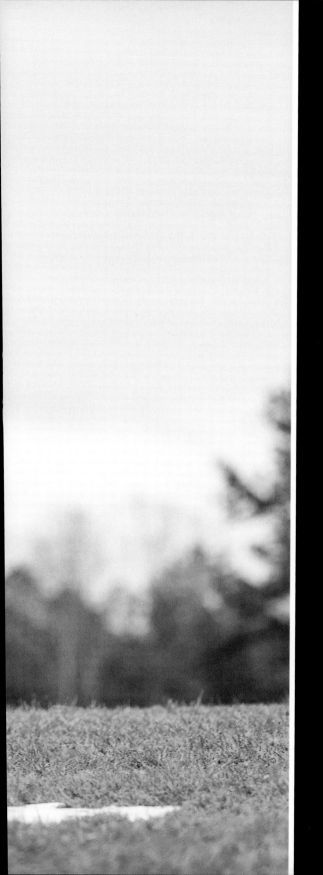

CHAPTER 3

OPEN UP TO NATURE

When I need a reset, the most powerful thing I can do to get myself grounded again is to take a walk in nature. It doesn't need to be the woods; it could be the water, the beach, the desert—anywhere that's quiet enough for me to hear birds and breeze more than cars and people.

It's hard to feel down when you're out in the natural world, and there's a reason for that. Scientists would call it quantum physics, but most of us call it vibes; it's the notion that everything in nature is made up of vibrations. Your body is essentially a tower of energy; trillions of atoms vibrating at a frequency that allows them to hold together in the shape of you. The higher your vibrating frequency, the more in touch you are with your higher power—whether you call that power God or Nature or however you want to look at it. The higher your vibrating frequency, the more positive you feel and more of a positive vibe you give off. Lower vibrations are associated with fear, depression, and anger.

Our own vibrations change in response to our environment, and the vibrations in nature are simply higher, and more positive, than those in the man-made world.

Think back to the last time you were in a really bad mood. Your thoughts were probably running toward the negative as well. That's because thoughts have energy. They don't come out of nowhere; your brain manufactures them and sends them out. Negative thoughts have a lower vibrational energy than positive thoughts, and that energy is reflected in the way you feel—your mood—and in the energy you put out to other people.

"Everything in life is vibration."

—ALBERT EINSTEIN

Have you ever felt immediately comfortable with someone, or walked into a home and felt at ease right away? That's the result of people putting out positive energy. We feel it from other people, but we often forget that others can feel energy coming from us as well. When you're putting out those positive vibes—and as I said earlier in this book, if you're not feeling so positive, then fake it!—you're going to put other people at ease, and attract the types of people and energy you want. People with similar energies attract one another. Your vibe attracts your tribe.

The Good-Vibes Workout

Almost every day, my workout begins with a brief exercise to calm my subgenual prefrontal cortex.

Never heard of that body part before? Me neither; I actually had no idea that I was doing this until I started working on this book. It was then that I came across some research on this obscure but powerful section of the brain.

The subgenual prefrontal cortex (sgPFC) is actually a part of the brain that's responsible for our self-image. When you're in a calm, positive place, this section of your mind is relatively quiet. But when it gets stimulated, you start to think negative thoughts about yourself. In other words, controlling the impulses in your brain is an essential part of any mind/body fitness plan.

And how do you do it? Simply by spending a little time in nature.

In 2015, researchers found that when people took walks in nature, then submitted to a brain scan, their sgPFC showed less activity, and the subjects reported fewer feelings of self-doubt. But when they took walks in an urban setting, they got no relief. Their brains were still shooting out sparks, and their thoughts were still running to the negative. Turns out the beauty of the natural world is a palliative against feeling sorry for ourselves.

That's something most of us know instinctively. To make the most of my time in the outdoors, sometimes I'll treat walking through nature as more of a moving meditation. I'll listen to something slow and positive like Rising Appalachia, Trevor Hall, Nahko, or East Forest (all worth checking out if you don't know them), or simply put on a Pandora station for yoga workout music. I'll think about the words or move with the music as opposed to just letting my mind wander.

I get a dose of nature almost every day because, to get to the gym on my property, I take a short hike up a hilly road that borders a woods filled with deer, hawks, and coyotes. Ella and Dallas usually come with me, because they love patrolling the open space, too.

I actually love that the gym is a half mile from the house because I get to spend time in nature—and I am getting the extra work on my sgPFC. Mental *and* physical workout!

Get Back to the Green

Most of us not only don't live in nature; we've done everything we can to expel it from our lives. I get it; spending time in nature means not engaging with society in a way that we've been taught is crucial to "getting ahead." That's true when it comes to our self-care as well. It's hard for me to set aside time for nature when my mind is nagging me to fit in another interval cardio or CrossFit workout. But it's something I have to make the effort to spend time with. I'm an Aries, which is a fire sign; I need to balance out that fire and energy with something calming and quiet.

"Be thankful for what you have; you'll end up having more. If you concentrate on what you don't have, you will never, ever have enough."

—OPRAH WINFREY

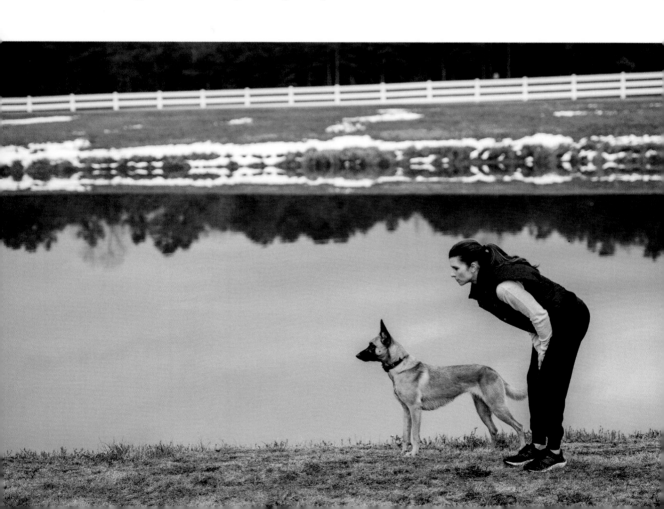

It's easier when I'm in North Carolina, but I also spend some time in my apartment in Chicago, and admittedly, the city has a lot to offer: great nightlife, museums, theater, depression, restaurants, culture . . .

Oh yeah, I sorta slipped that *depression* word in there. Studies show that living in the city increases one's risk for depression and other mental illnesses, in part because being divided from nature causes us to suffer repeated negative self-thought (that old low-frequency brain activity again). Surrounded by society, we stop seeing ourselves for what we truly are—a part of the great cycle of nature and life— and instead see ourselves as we imagine others might. We start to measure ourselves against other people, with a predictable result: compare and despair.

> "Comparison is the thief of joy."
> —THEODORE ROOSEVELT

Nature Makes You an Instant Success

When you think of what signifies success in society, it's money, fame, possessions—stuff we can never get enough of, because there will always be someone more famous, more wealthy, more successful. But success in nature? That means nothing more than fresh air, clean water, and a shady spot to rest your head. Once you have that, you have enough.

Nature helps us put our values back in place and to stop comparing ourselves to others. Nobody ever takes a deep breath of cool mountain morning and worries about whether somebody else has more fresh air than they have!

Nature Gets Your Creative Juices Flowing

One study found that people who spend time in nature perform up to 50 percent better on creative problem-solving tests. That makes sense to me: as much as I love working in my WOman cave, I get my inspiration from nature. Going outside helps me think of new directions and new ideas, instead of getting stuck mulling over the same old hassles and arguments in my mind.

If you don't have regular access to nature, consider bringing some indoors with you. One study found that when people stared at scenes of nature for ten minutes, they felt less stress when tackling difficult tasks than those who looked at images of man-made environments. But make your decorations dramatic: Hang some Ansel Adams posters on your wall. Make your screensaver a glorious waterfall. Another study found that those who looked at images of awe-inspiring natural landscapes got more stress relief than those who looked at photos of gardens or parks. Nature sounds have the same effect, so maybe when you're feeling stressed, try relaxing to the sound of babbling brooks instead of Garth Brooks. (To be clear, though, I do love Garth Brooks!)

"The Law of Attraction is all about vibration. Everything is vibrational, your thoughts, your ideas, every being. You will draw to you whatever vibration matches yours, wanted or unwanted."

—UNKNOWN

The Natural Vibes Wish List

In our busy lives, we often don't realize that nature can be a lot closer than we think. Even if you live in an urban center, a large park or a nearby suburban area can offer a natural respite. Start planning your escapes into nature, and start taking them regularly.

1. List three places within twenty minutes of your home where you can experience the vibes of nature today.

   _____

   _____

   _____

2. List three amazing places within five hours' drive where you can take a weekend to relax in nature.

   _____

   _____

   _____

3. List three natural wonders or national parks in the United States that you've always wanted to visit.

   _____

   _____

   _____

4. List three places anywhere in the world that would be your dream escape from civilization.

   _____

   _____

   _____

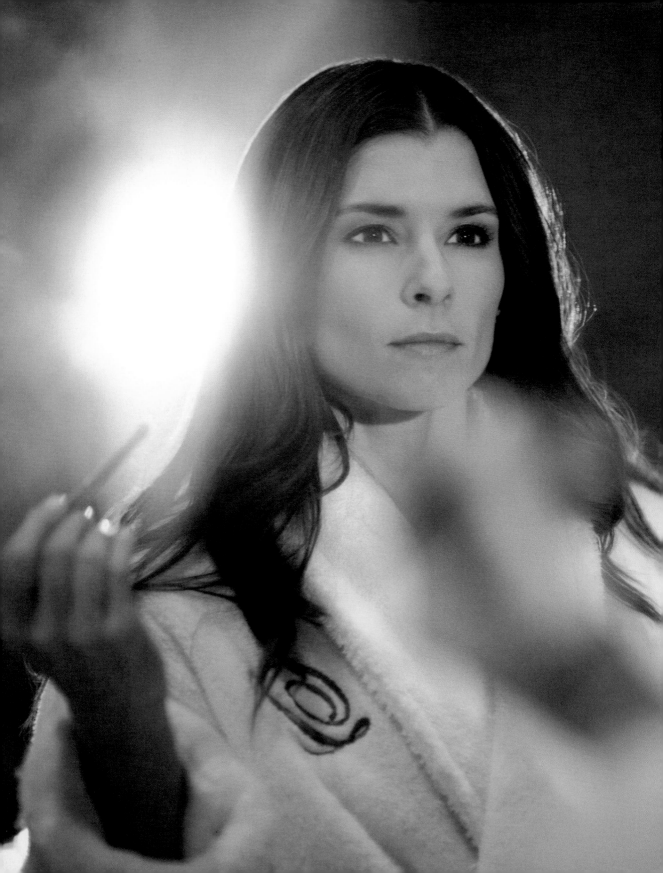

CHAPTER 4

DREAM BIG

Whenever I sign autographs for kids, I almost always sign them, "Dream Big!" But kids don't usually have trouble dreaming big. It's their parents who don't dare to dream big enough.

Kids always gravitate to the unlikely or the impossible. But as we get older, we begin to convince ourselves that circumstances, responsibilities, and our own personal shortcomings are too much to overcome. We bury our dreams under the excuses we tell ourselves in order to feel better about giving up.

Let's try to uncover those dreams once again.

Don't Be Afraid to Be Afraid

"If your dreams don't scare you, they're not big enough." That's a quote I think of often, from politician and writer Ellen Johnson Sirleaf.

The question I often ask myself and others is: "If you could do anything in your life, what would it be?" So many adults don't have an answer. (Kids almost always do!)

Do you have an answer? If not, why? Have you given up creating and chasing dreams? Are you just comfortable where you are today? Or have you just stopped believing big dreams are possible?

If you're working in your comfort zone—physically, emotionally, intellectually— then you're not going to grow, and your biggest dreams are going to stay far out of reach. You need to always be challenged by the tasks ahead of you and frightened by the possibility of actually reaching your goals. Look for a peak that's dizzyingly high. That's where you want to be headed.

Keep Taking the Next Step

If you had told me ten years ago that I'd be body-confident enough to be posing for photos like the one on the cover of this book, I'd have said you were nuts. I made that level of fitness my goal—that's why I've spent the past several years documenting my personal journey on Instagram and other social media outlets.

You and I are no different. I grew up in a very small town in Illinois and have insecurities just like the next person. Based on extensive trial and error and personal evolution,

> "I don't have a stomach pooch anymore. I'm even thinking I might wear a bikini this summer!"

JULIE GRUNWALD, 42
Charlotte, North Carolina

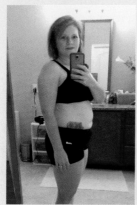

BEFORE   AFTER

"I thought I was working out, and I thought I was in pretty decent shape," says Julie. "I'd try spinning classes at the gym or group fitness classes. But then I took Danica's Fit Test and it really kicked my ass."

Discovering that she had so much room for improvement got Julie excited for the challenge. "I started gaining weight after my daughter was born, when I was thirty-five," she says. "I thought I was eating healthy, but every year I gained a couple of pounds." She even tried the Whole30 program, but flunked out twice: "It was so restrictive. I ran out of food to eat because it seemed like everything wasn't allowed."

But *Pretty Intense* kept her engaged with new workouts and new foods to try. "My husband bought me a spiralizer and I became obsessed with it. I started spiraling everything—zucchini, squash, sweet potatoes—and I absolutely love cauliflower rice. My family doesn't even notice the switch. It's great to have what looks like starch on your plate but in fact it's actually a vegetable and good for you. I keep it simple because I have a six-year-old to please, too."

But what Julie is most pleased with is her results. "The biggest change for me, and the one everyone comments on, is that my waist is very clearly defined now. I lost four and a half inches off my waist, almost two sizes in pants. I don't have a stomach pooch in front anymore. I'm even thinking I might get away with a bikini this summer.

"After about week seven or eight, the weight just started to fall off my body. And my butt looks really nice, too! Once you start to see those changes, you don't ever want to go back!"

my dream (one of them) is to help people create lifestyle goals and learn how to follow through with them.

I knew it would take time to get good at any challenge I put on myself, and I knew it would involve both successes and setbacks. (My earliest attempts at yoga poses look more like plane crash photos than yogi contentment.) But while I had a long-term goal, I also knew the path to that end result was a series of goals that I could set for myself and, yes, really achieve. Setting, and reaching, a goal gives me an ongoing sense of accomplishment.

That's how I set up the exercise portion of this book. You'll set a new goal each week. Many of them may become lifetime healthy habits. Others might not fit in with your overall lifestyle. But each time you succeed at reaching a new goal, you'll have taken another step up the ladder to your dream body and mind.

> "Don't let what you cannot do interfere with what you can do."
>
> —JOHN WOODEN

Thing is, this is the same approach you should take toward any enormously lofty goal, from owning your own business to getting a degree to resetting a relationship. Set your goals, then, every so often, take a moment to reflect on how you're doing. You'll be surprised at how many successes you've had, and you'll be able to more clearly see where you might have failed and how you can do better next time. Giant, seemingly impossible dreams become possible slowly, with little steps. But what we need is constant feedback and assurance that we're progressing toward them. That's what goals will give you.

Ask for What You Want

Most of us forget this simple step. If you're a believer, as I am, don't be afraid to ask God for what you want.

That doesn't mean praying for a million dollars to fall from the sky. It means stating out loud, to yourself and to God (although some would prefer to say "the universe"), what you want to achieve, and then asking for the personal strength, courage, and determination to go out and get it. You'll find that when you dare to pray out loud for your ambitions, you'll be more daring in your pursuit of them.

Asking for what I want—and asking for help in achieving it—helps me stay humble. Humility is a trait that, for most of us, takes work and practice. Admitting you don't have the power to achieve your goals alone, and asking God for help, takes a lot of the burden off your shoulders. You don't have to have a big ego to have big dreams. Ordinary people achieve extraordinary things every single day.

Remember that life changes fast. Situations—good ones and bad ones—don't last, and you're always going to be reevaluating what you want your life to look like. Maybe

"I'm full of energy—and I feel like I have a lot less stress!"

RICK NEUBERT, 65
Port St. Lucie, Florida

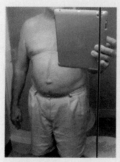 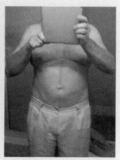

BEFORE   AFTER

A semi-retired patient coordinator, Rick still fast-walks his dogs six to seven miles a day. But all that cardio exercise wasn't making much of an impact. Then after just six weeks on *Pretty Intense*, he dropped twenty pounds and four inches from his waist.

"My clothes fit a lot better, and I just feel better overall," Rick reports. "I don't have to worry about what I'm wearing—'oh gosh, my stomach's sticking out!' In fact, I got rid of a whole bunch of clothes that I couldn't wear anymore—they were too big! I gave them to Goodwill."

Rick's goal was to slim down enough to fit into a favorite suit in time for his daughter's graduation. But in losing the pounds, he was surprised at all that he gained. "I was feeling lazy, even though I walked a lot. I'd get home from work and feel drained." But after starting *Pretty Intense*, his whole life turned around. "I'm full of energy. I don't sit around and watch TV much anymore. I go out a lot more, and I feel like I have less stress."

your biggest goal is a new job, or a new relationship, or changing the way you look and feel. Whatever it is, remember that your goals are, ultimately, between you and your higher power; those are the only two entities you need to impress. It's easier to achieve greatness when we don't feel like we have to prove ourselves to anybody else. Also, don't forget, we can do everything possible to plan our life, but we need to be ready for setbacks, changes, and challenges. Everything happens for a reason.

Forgive Yourself

I'm always telling myself that my primary goal is to be the best I can be *at this time*, and if I keep that as my focus, I'll always be okay with myself and where I am right now.

We all start out with our own unique liabilities. As I said earlier, keep in mind that we're all trying our best, pretty much all the time. If you fail—whether it's falling off your diet and workout plan, or something much more grave at work or in your personal relationships—don't fall into the common trap of thinking, "That's who I am; I'm always screwing up." Don't tell yourself that story; that's your mind river carving a path in the wrong direction.

You need to be willing to forgive yourself. But that's not always easy: we often find it easier to forgive others' mistakes than to forgive our own. So try this: Think back to a mistake you made that still haunts you. Now imagine that the person who screwed up is someone else, someone who was essentially doing the best they could at the time. Can you forgive *that* person? Of course you can. Forgive that person; that person is you. Hold on to the lessons you might have learned from your mistakes, but let go of everything else. Now!

You today are someone totally new.

> "To make the right choices in life, you have to get in touch with your soul. To do this, you need to experience solitude, which most people are afraid of, because in the silence you hear the truth and know the solutions."
>
> —DEEPAK CHOPRA

Worksheet: Big Dreams

Break your goals into these three categories and then list a few of the most important things to accomplish . . .

    1. Professionally

    _____

    2. Emotionally

    _____

    3. Spiritually

    _____

List five "bucket-list" activities you dream of one day accomplishing. They could be creative (write a screenplay), physical (run a half marathon), travel-related (climb Mount Kilimanjaro), or anything else you can think of. But remember: If the dream doesn't scare you, it's not big enough!

    1. _____

    2. _____

    3. _____

    4. _____

    5. _____

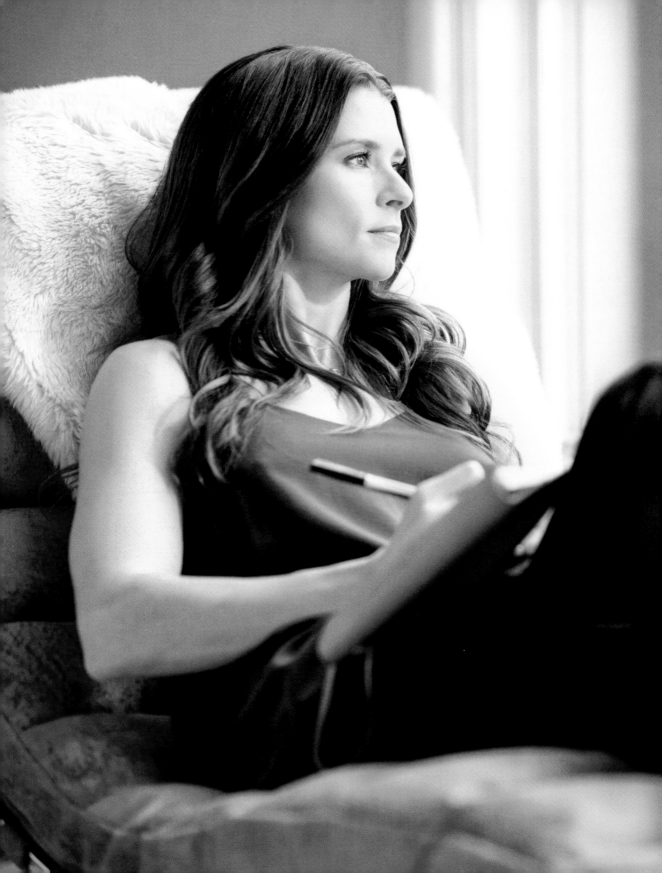

BECOME YOUR OWN BFF

One of the best things that has happened to me over the last few years of self-reflection and soul work is that I have learned how glorious it is to become my own best friend.

Being your own best friend is not the same as being self-centered or ego-driven, and it doesn't mean you get rid of your existing friends. In fact, the more of a friend you can be to yourself, the more you can give to others.

When you're dissatisfied with who you are, when you're uncomfortable with yourself, you tend to resent others for what you perceive they have. I have come to learn that our thoughts about others are in fact a reflection of *ourselves*. It's tough to recognize when it's happening, but it is so true. Every time we judge something or someone else, it's what we're judging about ourselves.

The old cliché—you can't love someone else until you first learn to love yourself—is really true. In fact, learning to fall in love with your own company, to be your own best friend, can be an enormous step toward having better relationships with others. Loving yourself means you have come to accept imperfections and learned to exercise patience for others, because that's what you are doing for yourself.

What does a best friend do? A best friend is there for you when you're down. A best friend acknowledges your feelings, forgives your mistakes, and lets you be whomever you really are. A best friend listens to your truth without judging you, and tells you the truth even if you don't want to hear it. A best friend empowers you to be the person you want to be. You never have to pretend to be someone else when you're with your best friend.

What a valuable lesson in life. When you are your own best friend, you don't *need* anyone or anything. You are good with the simpler things in life. You also have the confidence to be alone if that's what is best for you.

The question is, how do we get to that point?

Speak the Truth—Out Loud—to Yourself

You know how you get choked up when you try to express something truly important, something dramatic or serious or life-changing? You can live with a feeling stopped up inside of you for years, but say it out loud and suddenly it becomes real, and that can be scary.

> "Love yourself first and everything else falls into line."
>
> —LUCILLE BALL

That's why saying what's on your mind, out loud, is so important. Speak your own truth to yourself. Say, out loud, what you really want. *Say the words!* It's a critical step toward recognizing, and accepting, yourself and what truly motivates you. It's part of the process of learning about, and learning to love, yourself. The quicker you start admitting your truth, the quicker you become your own best friend. You begin to no longer need the approval or validation of someone else.

I must say, my WOman cave really helped with this process. It was a space where I could organically grow. The room had nothing in it, so all I did was start filling it up with items that brought me joy! And *only* those things. It provided me with constant feedback about my own priorities, my hopes and dreams and ambitions.

Have the Difficult Conversation

Once you have that level of respect for yourself, it becomes easier to give, and to get, respect from others.

We want people to like us, so we avoid confronting situations because it might make others not like us as much. But often, what we sacrifice in our efforts to get others' acceptance is their respect. And in the end, it's hard to really like someone you don't respect. Once you become your own best friend, once you can move beyond the need to please others, you'll find that you're having more honest and respectful relationships with friends, family, and coworkers.

One of the most respectful things you can do, both for yourself and the people in your life, is to confront conflicts head-on. I realize that's not as easy as it seems. For many of us, our very nature makes us want to avoid "the difficult conversation."

When I'm unhappy with the actions that someone is taking—whether it's my boyfriend or one of my girlfriends or someone I work with—I say so. I no longer swallow my feelings, and it has made all the difference in my relationships. When I used to hold things in, I'd get resentful. Those resentments would grow, and a strain would develop between me and the other person. Today my relationships are more open, more honest, and more fulfilling, because I'm direct with others, and I make it clear that it's okay for them to be direct with me.

Don't be afraid to confront a difficult situation; it usually goes a lot better than you think it will. Practice makes it easier. Keep it short, keep it sweet, make it respectfully honest. You'll gain the respect of others, but more important, you'll gain the respect of the person who matters most: yourself.

> "Just give yourself permission to tell the truth to yourself."
>
> —IYANLA VANZANDT

Soul Advice

Have you ever noticed that it's often easier to figure out the direction others should take than to decide on a direction for yourself? We don't wrestle with self-doubt when we're making decisions for others. That's why so many people are eager to give you advice. So why are we afraid to trust our own instincts?

In the end, only you will be responsible for your own happiness. So it makes sense that only *you* should be making the decisions that will determine whether or not you'll be happy. Your soul/heart/intuition—whatever you want to call it—knows you best. Develop a relationship with your all-knowing soul. All the advice you need is deep down inside *you*!

Detach from Outcomes

When you're always taking the next healthy step mentally and physically, you're as in charge of your life as you can be.

But what happens after you take that action—how others react to you, whether you get that job or that award or that opportunity—isn't something you're in charge of. Wallowing in "what ifs" doesn't do you any good; in fact, it's a distraction from taking the next positive, powerful, passionate step forward. Learn to trust that the universe has your back! When you look back at your life, I bet you can think of quite a few situations that happened, things that seemed like setbacks, but of which you can now say, "I'm so glad that happened!" Everything happens for a reason. I believe that with my whole heart.

Instead of thinking about "what ifs," think back to the Mind River chapter: your thoughts become your reality. The two most important actions I take for my well-being are detaching from outcomes—I take responsibility for doing my best, not for the end results—and following the path of least resistance.

"My body changed more than I thought was possible."

JENNA MORAN, 46
Bozeman, Montana

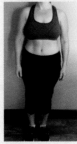 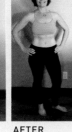

BEFORE   AFTER

After a long career in real estate, Jenna decided to make a lifestyle change and got her degree in interior design. She wanted to make other changes, as well: After a going on a diet and dropping fifteen pounds, she wanted to up her fitness level. *Pretty Intense* not only did that, but it stripped another ten pounds of unwanted fat from her body.

What worked for Jenna was not just the variety of exercises—which she could do alone in her basement at any hour she liked—but the motivation of knowing that she had a community of people working out with her. "I was a full-time student, so there were days that I didn't get the workouts in until late in the night, but the format and flexibility helped to keep me accountable and motivated to get it done, even if I was tired."

The result: "My body changed more than I thought was possible in that amount of time. It feels really good to feel good in my body. I look leaner, and seeing the changes in size and the way clothes fit was more exciting than stepping on the scale. I love it when I catch a glimpse in the mirror and think, 'Oh, look at that!,' as opposed to getting a glimpse of something that I'm not excited about."

Be the Light

I follow the Golden Rule, the same one they teach in Sunday school: Act toward others the way you'd like them to act toward you. Be a force for positivity. Don't latch on to your negative feelings, your stress and your fears and your anger. Be that person who walks into a room or up to someone and makes them smile. Bring others up to your high-vibin', happy, grateful level of light. It starts with a smile, then eye contact, an open heart, and respect . . . You might be just what that person needs that day.

This isn't easy to do—it's one of those behaviors that takes daily, conscious practice—but it will help to direct you along a path to achieving your goal of becoming your own best friend. How? Because when you treat others with kindness, it becomes easier to treat yourself that way, too. This isn't as easy as it sounds. Most of us hit days when we're cranky, irritable, and focused more on our own well-being than the feelings of others. Refocusing on improving the lives of those around us is one of the best ways to overcome those feelings, and that refocus will pay off. This is where mantras come in real handy!

"Every cell in your body is eavesdropping on your thoughts."

—DEEPAK CHOPRA

I think of it as self-esteem cleaning: when I take time to see the good in other people, that's when I feel closest to the good inside of me.

Vision Board:
Get to Know Your New Best Friend

Take a moment to scroll through the pictures on your phone or camera. Write down, in categories, what you take pictures of. For example, I have a lot of pictures of dogs, nature, yoga, food, clothes, workout ideas, sweaty exercise selfies, my boyfriend, my family.

_____

_____

_____

_____

Taking stock of what you capture most in your own life will give you a new perspective on what's of greatest value to you. And it will clue you in to what you might be missing, and needing more of, in your life.

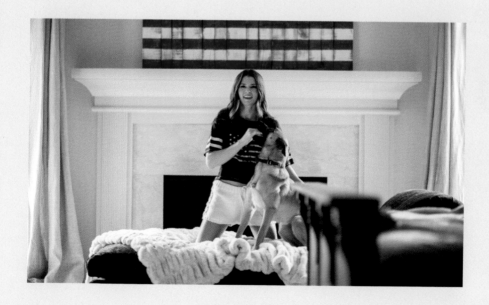

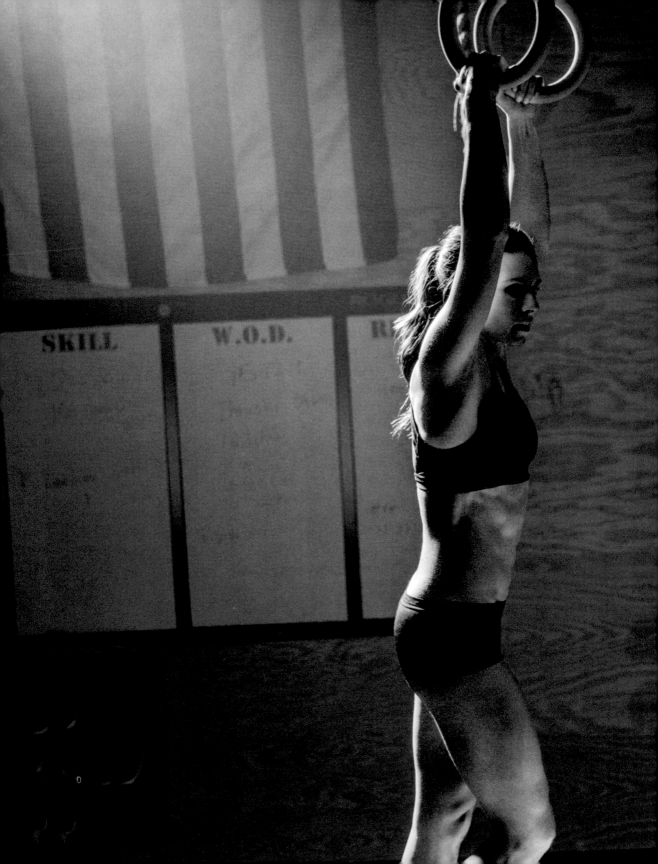

PART TWO

The *Pretty Intense* Body

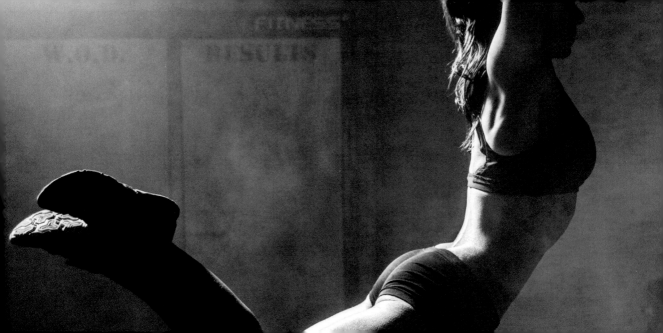

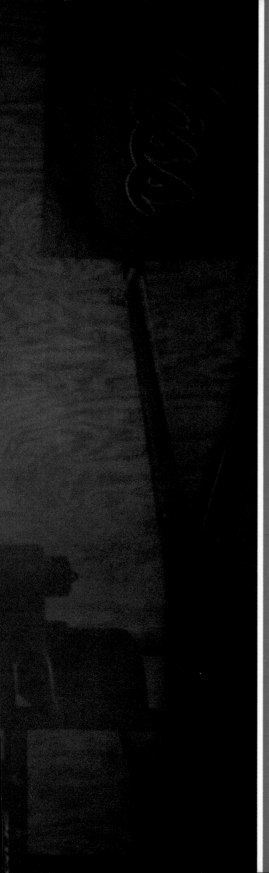

CHAPTER 6

PAIN IS MENTAL—
I PROMISE!

Intensity is a principle that has guided and informed me throughout every aspect of my life. Living a *Pretty Intense* life means living to the fullest, body and mind, every single day. I try to do everything with intensity—meaning without distraction, without self-focused doubt or fear, without the need to seek approval from others.

The first part of this book was designed to help you capture that mind-set, to bring your dreams and aspirations into focus and help you carve a path toward realizing them. Bring that intensity to your career, your relationships, your hobbies, your entire life. The perspectives and tools you discovered in the first few chapters will help you become stronger above your shoulders.

Having a clear set of goals for your life is the first step toward improving your physical fitness. If you don't feel like your life is on the right path, it's going to be hard to dedicate yourself to a workout program and stick to it; when you doubt yourself, you doubt your decisions and your choices. No wonder it becomes easy to question whether you need to go to the gym today, or to cheat when the workout starts to get tough.

So building mental and emotional intensity and intention is the first step. That is why you did so many exercises to test your hopes, dreams, and mental and emotional dedication. This chapter is about bringing that intense mind-set into your workouts— to start building strength and endurance below the shoulders, too.

These are the tricks I use to push through tough workouts and keep myself motivated to hit the gym each day.

It's Hard to Work Your Ass Off, But It Works Your Ass Off

Have you ever gone to the gym and seen people marching along on a treadmill or stair climber while watching the TV? Or sitting on a bench doing wrist curls while chatting up a cute member of the opposite sex? Maybe that person was you.

That's a fine way to burn an hour or so, but it's not going to burn very much fat. It's not going to make you stronger, sculpt your body into the shape you want it, or build overall health and endurance. It's not a workout. Exercising with distractions is not exercising with intensity, and it's unlikely you'll see the results you truly seek. Workouts

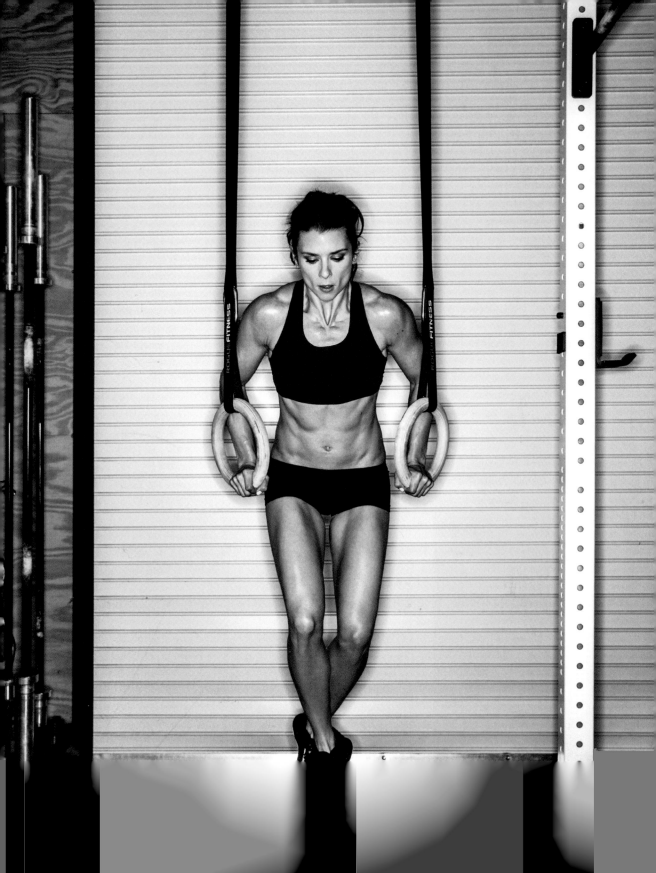

> "Don't get too comfortable with who you are at any given time—you might miss the opportunity to become who you want to be."
>
> — JON BON JOVI

are work. Otherwise, they'd be called chill-outs. That's what I do when I walk the dogs.

And the success of a workout can't be measured by how long it took you or how much sweat you pumped out. It's measured by real progress—how much longer you can sustain your effort, how much more you can lift, how much faster you can go—and by how much of the time you spend outside your comfort zone.

Get Comfortable with Discomfort

The bottom line is this: If you want to get in shape you are going to have to push past your comfort zone, all the time. Yes, you will still burn calories doing something that doesn't make you feel like you want to lie down on the floor at the end of a workout (which I do about half the time, by the way), but you won't achieve what you really want. I am guessing what you really want is a lean, strong, and well-performing machine.

Your mind is a very powerful thing, and it's going to be your biggest weapon in your quest to look and feel amazing. The key is to convince yourself you can handle it (because, yes, you can!). The more confident you are stepping outside your comfort zone, the more comfortable you'll be with discomfort. Here are some common ways your mind will try to go rogue on you, and how to bring it back into line so you can keep heading toward what you want.

———

THE PAIN: Feeling as if you just don't want to exercise today.

PUSH PAST IT: Remind yourself about the last successful workout you had. Remember how strong and in command you felt afterward. Drive toward capturing that feeling again.

MANTRA: *I will thank myself when I'm done.*

THE PAIN: Feeling frustrated or exhausted, like you want to quit in the middle.

PUSH PAST IT: Remind yourself *why* you're working this hard: Go back to the goals and dreams you filled out on pages 65 and 85.

MANTRA: *If I want something I've never had, I am going to have to do something I've never done.*

———

THE PAIN: Feeling like you're pushing yourself too far—you're too uncomfortable.

PUSH PAST IT: Emotionally detach. Most exercise pain is mental, not physical, so try to absorb the pain as nothing more than information— because that's exactly what it is. It's information telling you you're moving toward your goal.

MANTRA: *What doesn't kill me makes me stronger.*

Slow Down, But Don't Stop

I tell people all the time when we are working out together that it's not as hard to just keep going as it is to stop . . . and have to talk yourself into starting again. It is something you'll get better at over time, but you have to keep pushing to reach new levels. As your strength and fitness grow rapidly, so will your body and mind both change to accept amazing new levels of endurance; your comfort zone will become greater.

Your job is to not accept that.

Try to be as ambitious as possible with each workout. It's better to overreach and run out of steam than it is to finish and say, "I could have gone harder" or (my favorite) "It wasn't that hard." *Every* workout can be hard if you go as fast as you can. Don't argue. It's true.

I try to make every workout I do as tough as possible, writing out my plan on a big whiteboard in my home gym. In fact, I tend to overprogram myself and have to go

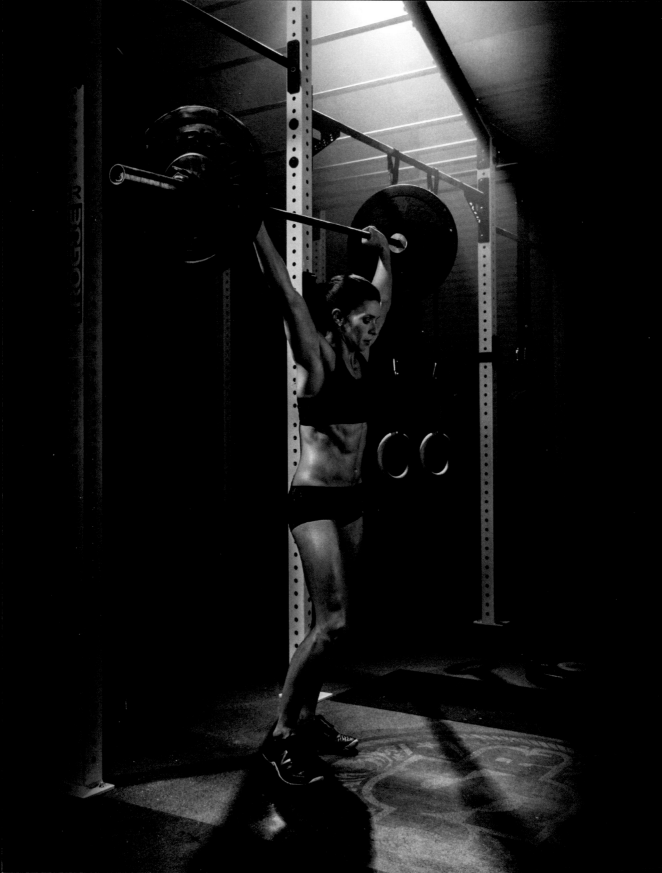

back to the whiteboard during the workout and drop the sets or reps. But the point is, I want every day that I take the time to train to be great and meaningful! If I half-ass my workout, I will get half the ass I want, ha-ha!

Give Yourself a Boost

I have up days and down days. Sometimes I feel strong, sometimes I feel as if I could sprint in the Olympics, and sometimes I feel like I suck. I also have days when I'm very busy and need to push through a workout as quickly as possible. So I have to come up with tricks to help get through the workout as fast and efficiently as possible. Here are seven tricks I use to help dig deeper and get more out of myself.

1. **Use a timer.** I very rarely work out without timing the workout duration or using it as a countdown for the length of time I want to work. I recommend one with a beeper or a countdown so it triggers a "go time" response in your mind.

2. **Record your results.** There is no reason you should take the time to work out and not write down your reps or time. It holds you accountable.

3. **Need the break.** That should be your mantra with any workout you do, especially interval-style workouts. Intervals will have set breaks to let you rest and recover, but your job is to push yourself as hard as you can toward that break. If you don't need the one-minute break, or whatever is in the workout plan, when it comes around . . . you're not working hard enough.

4. **Time your stops.** When you are in the middle of a workout and have to stop . . . do it. But give yourself a certain number of seconds and then get going again. I try to limit my stops to a five count.

5. **Own your form.** When your form starts to break down, and you find yourself cheating on moves, you're no longer doing the workout. Don't mistake movement for progress; you don't get any credit for squeezing in five more push-ups if you only got halfway down. That's true of any exercise—especially the ones that involve weights. When you cheat on form, you cheat yourself. Plus, you put your joints at

risk of injury, and nothing will knock you off your fitness game like time in rehab. Own your form: the only one around who can judge you is you.

6. Find your count. Sometimes doing fifteen reps can seem hard or boring, but doing five reps three times in a row seems somehow easier. Sometimes counting from one to fifteen can make you feel tired because it just emphasizes how much work you've already done, but counting from fifteen down to one points out how little work you have ahead of you, and keeps you motivated and your energy up. Play around with how you count your reps, and you may find a technique that works especially well for you. It also helps you recognize your progress. As an example, I used to do sets of five push-ups; now I do ten.

7. Run your race. I think about this whether I am in the car or in the gym. It is important to learn how hard is hard for you. If you can do a workout without stopping, push a little harder. If you are spending more time trying not to keel over, dial it back. But you and only you know if you are stopping because you are lazy, or because you actually are pushing hard enough to consider the workout *Pretty Intense*.

Good Pain, Bad Pain

When you work out in a *Pretty Intense* way, your muscles are going to be sore; sometimes while you're working out, and for sure the day after. Sometimes a fun case of DOMS (delayed-onset muscle soreness) happens on day 2 and lasts for a few more after that. There's nothing wrong with that. But what's important to realize is the difference between muscle pain and tendon or ligament pain. Tendons connect muscle to bone; ligaments connect bones to one another. Neither of these benefit from overwork. In fact, overworking these connective tissues is a great way to set your workout back for months.

The telltale sign is joint pain. If your biceps are sore, great. If your elbows or wrists are sore, on the other hand, that means you were lifting too much weight, did too many reps, or cheated some of the reps. Sharp pain deep inside the shoulder, at the front or back of the knee, in the hips, or in the ankle, wrist, or elbow may signal a problem. The telltale signs are always in the joints.

Worksheet: Fitness Goals

I'm thrilled to have had the chance to share the mental and emotional strategies that have brought me personal happiness and success, and that have helped form the foundation on which I've built my fitness platform. But if you've made it this far, no doubt you're itching to get more in-depth with the workouts and eating plan. I'm excited for us to begin this fitness journey together!

What I've emphasized throughout this book is the importance of setting small, achievable goals for yourself and working toward them day by day, knocking them out as you progress. But at the same time, it's important to *dream big*! And here's your chance to do so.

On this page, I want you to write down five fitness goals you have for yourself. Before you start writing, let me offer some advice:

- **Try to be as specific as you can be.** You may want to "get back in shape," but that's pretty vague. How will you know when you get there? "Lose two inches off my waist" or "Be able to do a pull-up" or "Run a 10K" are all goals you can measure and achieve.

- **Don't focus on your weight.** This program is going to help you reshape your body by adding lean, firm muscle and burning off fat. But muscle weighs more than fat, and you may not see the same changes on the scale that you see in the mirror. Weight isn't a particularly good measure of your fitness, or your look. (In fact, you may actually gain a couple of pounds in the early stages as your body gets stronger and prepares to burn off flab.)

- **Consult your doctor.** Standard cautions apply: you should always consult your doctor before taking on a new diet or fitness plan. But a doctor can also give you numbers that will solidly measure your health and show your progress. This program should have a measurable effect on your blood pressure, heart rate, cholesterol, and blood glucose levels. And while mirrors can lie, blood tests don't.

1. _____

2. _____

3. _____

4. _____

5. _____

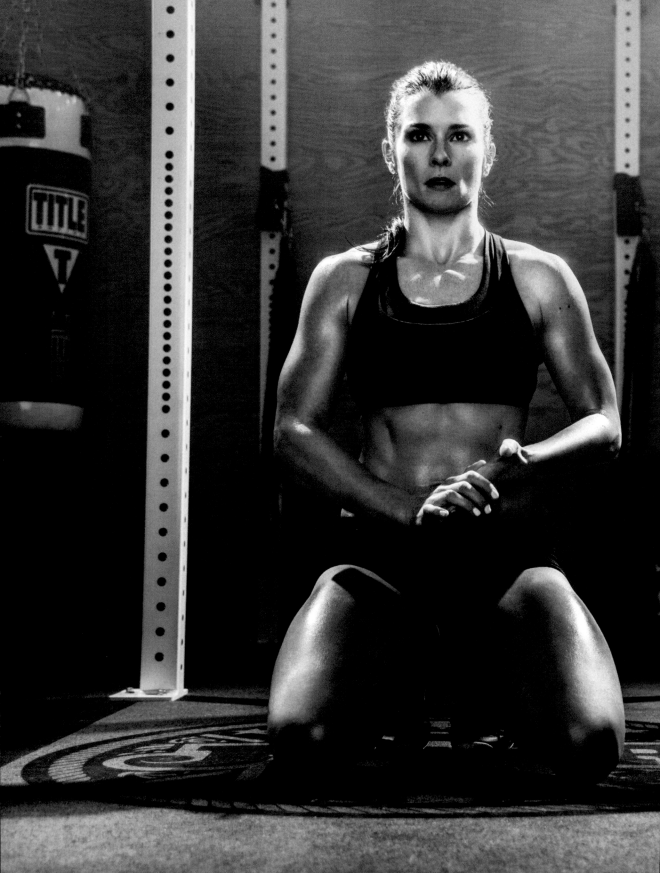

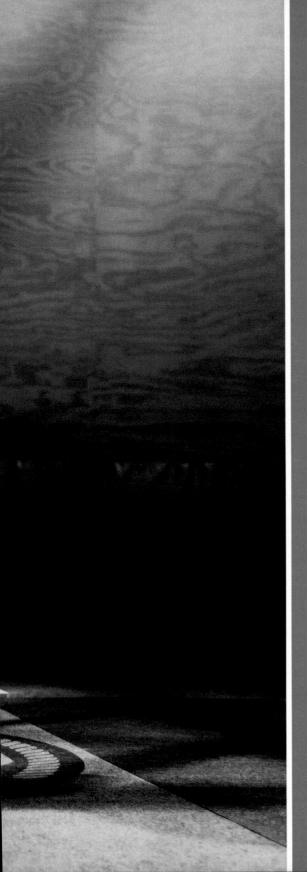

CHAPTER 7

MANTRAS WORK

When I was in sixth grade, one of my teachers had a poster on the wall that read *Carpe Diem*. I remember not knowing what that meant.

One day I asked, and once I understood what it meant, I would glance at that poster every day, and it started sinking in: *Seize the Day!*

Since then, mantras have been my thing.

I use mantras to motivate me, to calm me, to keep me focused. A mantra can be anything: a motivational saying, a couple of meaningful words, a prayer. If you've ever taken a yoga class and chanted "*Om*" at the end of it, that's a mantra. If you've said "Amen" in church or prayed before bedtime, that's a mantra. If you've ever told yourself "You can do this" before a big moment, that's a mantra, too.

Mantras can do a lot of things, but the primary thing they can do is help you focus—whenever you sense yourself overthinking a challenge, revving up an excuse, or are uncertain of what the next right move might be. You can use one of mine, make up your own, or grab an inspirational quote that keeps you focused when you're starting to waver. Mantras are the "smart bombs" of success; you can drop them right into your trouble zone and, boom, the trouble goes away.

Relax, Rinse, Repeat . . .

Even if you've never taken a yoga class or listened to a motivational speaker, chances are you've been repeating mantras since you were a child.

The most common form of mantra is prayer. We may say grace before dinner not just to express thanks, but to let go of the stress of the day and refocus ourselves on our home and family. We may say our prayers before bedtime not just to secure our relationship with God, but to help us relax and find sleep. If you've ever prayed for rain for your garden or sun for your softball game, you've been relieving stress by turning fate over to a higher power. That's a mantra.

You've also been doing something else, according to scientists: you've been pumping up your brain cells. One study found that after eight weeks of practicing a daily mantra, patients showed significant decreases in depression, insomnia, and pain. And in 2014, researchers did an extensive review of studies and found that repeating mantras or prayers reduced heart rate and blood pressure, decreased respiratory rates, reduced levels of stress hormones, and improved blood flow and oxygen flow to a part of the brain called the anterior cingulate cortex.

The anterior cingulate cortex is a part of the brain that helps to regulate heart rate and other unconscious functions of your body. It also plays a role in impulse control, emotions, and decision-making, and it seems to play a role in detecting errors; it lights up when something's amiss. In other words, if you want to calmly make smart decisions and be in charge of your life, this is the brain matter you want functioning at its highest possible level.

So the first use of mantras is to let go of stress so that we can enjoy not just better physical health, but better emotional health as well. And that leads, naturally, to better decision making. Something as simple as "Let it go" when you feel resentment or unwanted thoughts coming into your head can completely change your perspective just when you need it most.

Stop Thinking, Start Doing

How often do you hear someone explain a screw-up or a lapse in judgment with the excuse "I wasn't thinking"? A lot, I bet, but I'm going to propose an alternate way of looking at our mistakes: most of us screw up not because we're thinking too little, but because we're thinking too much.

After all, if your regular workout is at six P.M. and you choose not to go, chances are you probably came up with a well-thought-out excuse: "I'm too tired." "I can't fit it in." "My legs hurt." Standing up, putting on your gear, and starting to work out takes little, if any, thought at all. It's figuring out why you can't go that requires some real thinking. (The same goes for breaking your diet. Once you've settled on your food choices and decided to stick by them, they'll become automatic. It takes a little bit of thinking to go, "Oh, it's okay to have the M&M's because . . .")

In auto racing, as in any sport, there are times when you need to be thinking and times when you need to let go of active thinking and let your

> "Don't give up what you want the most for what you want right now."
>
> —UNKNOWN

body react to situations as they unfold. The same is true when you're working out; learning to trust your body and let go with your mind is an important skill in any sort of athletics.

This is where a mantra can be incredibly effective. When I'm pushing myself to the max in the gym and I feel as if I want to quit, my go-to mantra is "Slow down, don't stop." I don't have to think about the importance of continuing my workout or talk myself out of the way I feel. I just throw down that mantra and push through.

"I gave myself a present for my sixtieth birthday— a body I can be proud of!"

JAYNE GAUCI, 60
Indianapolis, Indiana

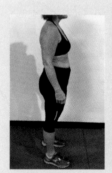

BEFORE   AFTER

"I've always been chunky," says Jayne. "Most of my adult life I've been over 175 pounds. When my sixtieth birthday approached, I decided, 'All my life I've been taking care of everyone else. What do I want for my sixtieth? I want something I've never had: a body I can be proud of.'"

When Jayne heard about the *Pretty Intense* Challenge, she told her personal trainer, who pooh-poohed the idea that someone her age could get fit by following my workout. "Danica Patrick is a professional athlete," the trainer scoffed. So Jayne fired the trainer, and started to chase her new goal.

And the result? "I weigh less now than I did in high school," she says. "But mostly I feel like I've turned the clock back twenty years on my body. The thing I didn't like about getting older was that I had lost my waistline. Now I have this amazing waist, and I can wear a belt."

But it's not just the eleven pounds Jayne dropped that excites her; it's the muscle she gained. "My upper body is my pride and joy," she says. "The fact that I have amazing definition and my triceps are solid and I have these shoulders that are cut—I didn't think it was possible!"

Mantras = Motivation

Like I said, my first understanding of the power of mantras came with *Carpe Diem*, and I try to seize each and every day. That doesn't mean being a control freak or trying to bend the world to my will. It simply means that I'm determined to take all the opportunities that the day is presenting me with and make the most of them. If it comes to you, conquer it.

Here are some of the motivational mantras that work for me:

What doesn't kill you makes you stronger.

This too shall pass.

Fake it till you make it.

Dig deeper.

Try harder.

Tough times don't last; tough people do.

Love never fails.

Finish like a pro.

Suck it up, buttercup.

Dream big.

I could go on and on. These mantras and many others have been powerful tools for me in keeping a positive attitude and getting through tough days. And while you're welcome to steal anything in this book and use it as a mantra, remember that what's between these covers is what works for me. Your goal is to find what works for *you*!

Worksheet:
Your Magic Mantra Maker

There are a million mantras out there, and just googling "motivational mantras" will give you endless ideas to play with. But only you can truly know what matters most to you.

This exercise will help you find mantras that touch on your goals and core values. First, write out some keywords that are important to you. I've broken them down into three categories:

ACTION WORDS: These describe in general terms the action that you are taking. Sometimes that action doesn't sound like an action as all ("relax," "accept"), but in fact stepping back and letting things happen can be the hardest thing to do—and, often, the most valuable.

EXAMPLES: relax, work, fight, try, accept, allow, open, let go, dream, embrace, do, seek, love, forgive

VALUE WORDS: These describe what's sacred to you. They're the core values that you need to be mindful of when you're connecting the action to the goal.

EXAMPLES: God, spirit, nature, family, love, heart, friends, dedication, honesty, hope, generosity, truth, sincerity, kindness, forgiveness, respect

GOAL WORDS: These describe what you're shooting for. They can be specific ("Drop ten pounds") or general ("Look great"), but in general they're broad, thought-provoking words or ideas.

EXAMPLES: wealth, success, fame, victory, big, improve, strong, lean, health, power, mental strength, confidence, self-love, joy, awareness

Circle the words that mean the most to you. This is a great starting point for surfing the web to look for full quotes that include those keywords. Then write the full quotes in the space here . . . and anywhere else you want to be reminded of them. Maybe get a chalkboard so you can rotate them and write down new ones as you evolve!

ACTION: _____

VALUE: _____

GOAL: _____

MANTRA: _____

ACTION: _____

VALUE: _____

GOAL: _____

MANTRA: _____

ACTION: _____

VALUE: _____

GOAL: _____

MANTRA: _____

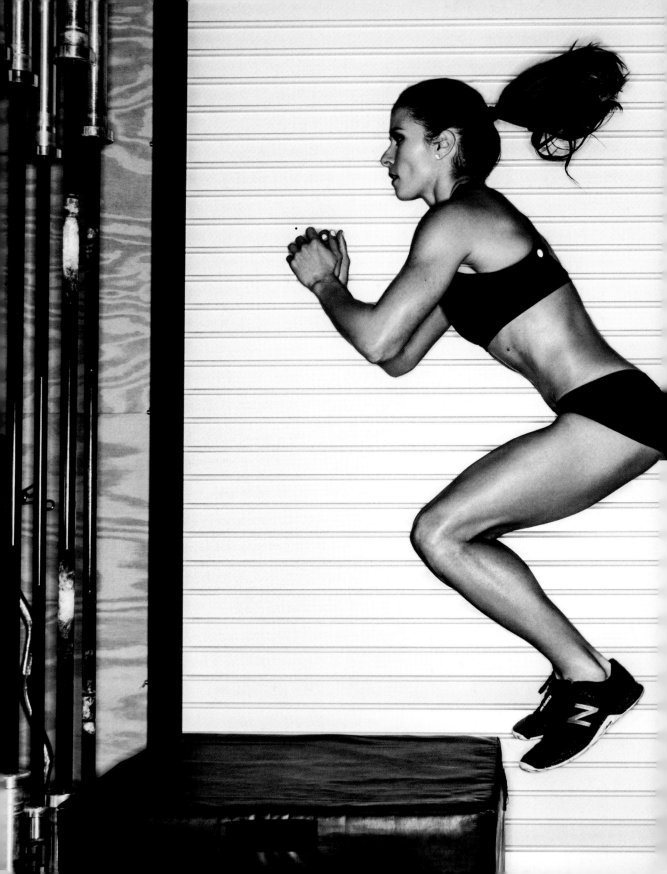

CHAPTER 8

INTENSITY!

As I said earlier, if you had told me ten years ago that I'd be posting photos of myself on Instagram in belly-baring workout gear, I would have said you were nuts. A decade ago I was exercising a lot, but I wasn't particularly happy with the way I looked. I was running thirty to forty-five minutes every single day and doing yoga a couple times a week, but I didn't look like I spent a ton of time working out. I had a small frame, but no muscle definition. I was 95 pounds and didn't look all that great. Now I weigh about 110 pounds and look far fitter!

Back then, I never really thought about the level of intensity I was putting into my workouts. It was more about how long I went, or how far I could go without stopping.

At the time, I was driving Indy cars, and I realized that I needed to develop more strength to help me handle them. I got a personal trainer who taught me that building muscle through resistance training would not only make me stronger, but would burn fat far more effectively than cardio. Once I started lifting weights, I also started looking like I went to the gym, and I finally had some muscle tone!

Nowadays the only running I do is short, fast, challenging, all-out intervals followed by a short walk recovery, repeated fifteen to twenty times. I know that learning about one's body is an ongoing process, and it takes trial and error to figure out what truly works for you—but man, I was way off for a long time!

The lesson of this chapter, then, is this: If you've ever felt like exercise just didn't work for you, or that you were putting in too much effort and not seeing results, or that you couldn't stick to a workout plan because you're not motivated enough, or because you're too stressed and too busy, I can almost guarantee that you're wrong. The problem isn't time, effort, or motivation. It's intensity. You need to work hard enough to be great.

Intervals and Intensity

High-intensity interval training, or HIIT, is the primary force behind my workouts nowadays. HIIT refers simply to a workout in which you go hard, at maximum intensity, for a certain amount of time, then back off for a "recovery" period before going at it hard again. You can do a HIIT workout with weights, on a bike, in a pool, on a treadmill—basically, whatever your favorite type of exercise, you can modify it to create an interval approach.

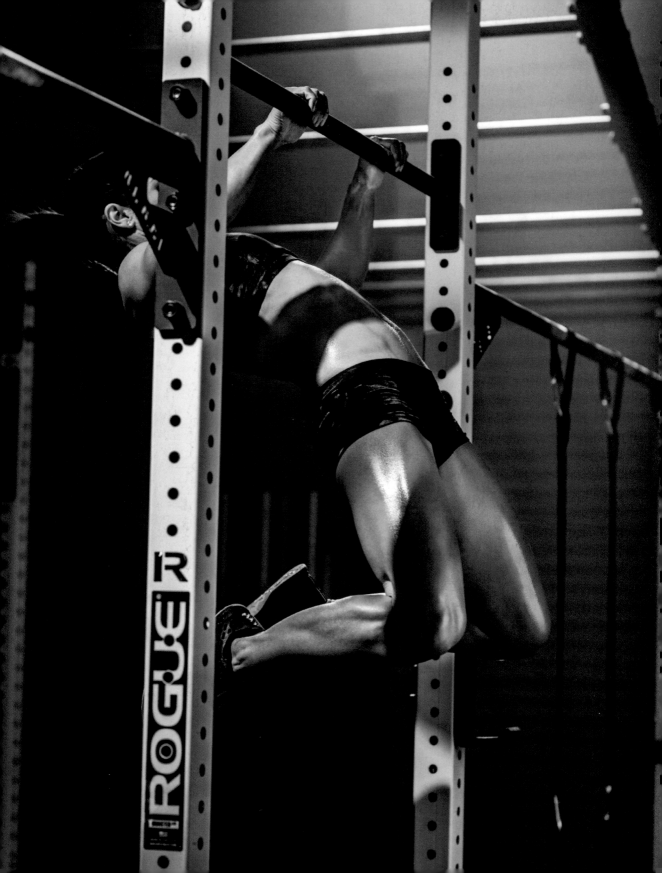

> "In any given moment we have two options: to step forward into growth or to step back into safety."
>
> —ABRAHAM MASLOW

What got me started on interval training was joining CrossFit. CrossFit is a style of workout that combines aerobic exercise, calisthenics (like push-ups and burpees), and weight lifting. You can do it alone, in a class, or as part of a team, which can be a ton of fun: my first CrossFit class was a Saturday team workout, and we won! (Given my competitive nature, I was into Cross-Fit hook, line, and sinker from day one.)

CrossFit workouts can vary widely; you can use published workouts or create your own by stringing together series of exercises. After we built our own CrossFit-style gym at the house, I started writing my own programming, and I have had a lot of fun writing some hybrid CrossFit/cross-training/HIIT workouts.

Burn, Baby, Burn

There's a lot to love about HIIT, but from a physical perspective, it's all about fat burning. When I was running an hour a day, I was skinny, but most of my weight loss came from muscle, not from fat. Burning calories is *not* the same as burning fat!

For example: Those cardio machines that show you when you're in the "fat-burning zone"? Total bullshit. Even the National Institutes of Health (NIH) has said, "The effect of regular aerobic exercise on body fat is negligible." (That's how you can get "skinny fat"—you lose weight, but much of the weight you lose is actually muscle, not fat!)

And while you might be burning calories while you're pedaling a bike or marching up a set of stairs, how long can you do that for? Twenty minutes? An hour? I don't want to be burning fat twenty minutes a day. I want to be burning fat 1,440 minutes a day. (And by the way, each of us has a unique metabolism that burns calories at our own pace; no machine can accurately tell us how many calories we're burning while we're on it.)

Too many of us work out all the time without seeing results, because the workouts we're doing simply aren't effective at boosting our metabolism. Burning calories on the stair climber or running on the roadway will shrink you a little, but it won't help you reshape your body. It won't give you a flat belly, sleek thighs, strong arms, and a tight, firm butt.

The *Pretty Intense* Workout will. It brings intensity back into your life, resetting your metabolism with brief, high-energy workouts that will program your body to burn the maximum amount of fat—not just when you're working out, but all day long. As you reset your internal calorie furnace with a combination of body-weight exercises, resistance training, and aerobic conditioning, you'll begin to see results on an almost daily basis.

Why You Can't Miss with HIIT

HIIT burns fat, builds muscle, improves both your aerobic fitness and your strength, and lowers your risk of obesity and diabetes by improving the way your body manages insulin. When your whole body is working hard, it recruits so much more muscle, and that really elevates your heart rate (building greater overall fitness). It also releases epinephrine and norepinephrine, two hormones that increase our physical energy, enhance fat burning, improve blood flow to the brain and muscles, and improve both memory and mental sharpness. Here's just a sampling of research that's been done on HIIT over the last decade:

- **HIIT releases your "bliss compound."** While scientists still debate the exact source of "exercise high," we know that intense training can release a brain chemical called anandamide, which is similar to compounds found in two other notorious sources of pleasure: chocolate and marijuana.

- **HIIT burns fat faster.** These hormones cause our fat cells to give up their precious stores so the fat within can be burned for energy (a process known as lipolysis). One review of studies found that HIIT was better at burning both subcutaneous fat (the stuff of love handles, saggy arms, and a junky trunk) and visceral fat (the stuff inside your belly).

- **HIIT builds endurance,** and it does it better than "endurance training." In a study of healthy young and middle-aged people, HIIT increased their VO_2 max levels (a measure of endurance) significantly more than longer, steady-state workouts.

- **HIIT protects you from diabetes.** Researchers looked at the effects of continuous exercise versus HIIT on insulin resistance and found that HIIT was more effective at reducing diabetes risk.

- **HIIT builds muscle and keeps you young.** An all-out sprint for just thirty seconds can raise your levels of human growth hormone (HGH) for up to two hours afterward, according to one study. HGH is the antiaging hormone: it improves your body's ability to burn fat and build muscle.

- **HIIT gets the job done faster.** Another study followed two groups of people for twelve weeks. One group did interval training for ten minutes a day, three times a week; the other did moderate-intensity training for forty-five minutes a day, three times a week. At the end of the study, the groups had similar improvements in both endurance and insulin resistance—despite the HIIT group working out more than one hundred minutes fewer each week!

- **HIIT makes you happier and less stressed.** Researchers at the University of Missouri-Columbus found that women who exercised at high intensity levels showed greater decrease in stress levels at thirty, sixty, and ninety minutes post-exercise than those who exercised at a more moderate rate.

- **HIIT is just more fun**, and you don't have to take my word for it: a study found that participants ranked HIIT (going all out for sixty seconds, then recovering for sixty seconds) as "more enjoyable" than steady-state moderate workouts.

> "Whether you think you can or you think you can't, you're right."
>
> —HENRY FORD

That last study doesn't surprise me at all. It is fun to push your body to see how far it can really go . . . and it's so much further than what you think. This is the second awesome component, besides fitness, that you'll get from HIIT: confidence! When you "kill" a workout, you feel on top of the world! You believe you can do anything. The more you do to build yourself up, the better for you and the better for the rest of your world.

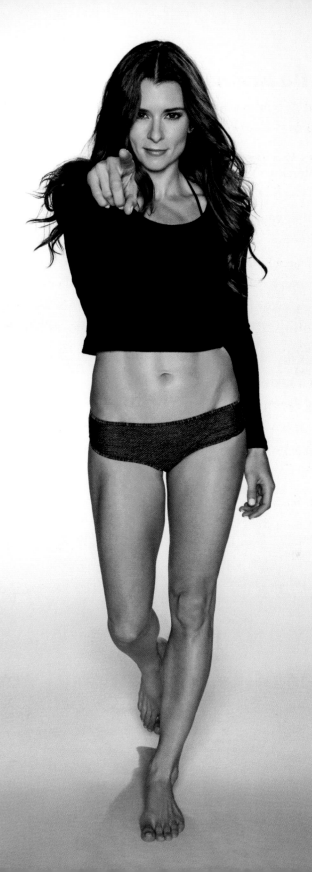

Dare to Be Intense!

Intensity is the key to getting greater results from everything you set your mind to, inside and outside the gym. Intensity comes in two forms:

- **Physical intensity.** The *Pretty Intense* Workouts require you to keep challenging your body. You'll move quickly; you'll lift challenging weights; you'll huff and puff and sweat. But you'll also be in and out of the gym much faster—and change your body much more quickly and effectively—than ever before. Too many of us waste time with long and unnecessary rest periods; with slow, steady cardio that doesn't have a real impact; with light weights that don't challenge our muscles or bring us results. (How many times have you seen some guy sitting on a bench at the gym doing wrist curls? Ridiculous!) Remember: Work hard enough to be great.

- **Mental intensity.** An effective workout engages your mind just as much as it engages your body. Sitting on a stationary bike watching *Dr. Phil* while you pedal along does more than waste your time; it wastes your mental energy as well. Exercise is active. When you're exercising with intensity, you're constantly monitoring your movements:

Is my form correct for each repetition?

Am I pushing myself as hard as I can?

Am I listening to my body?

Do I know the next exercise I'm moving to?

You can't answer those questions if you're busy listening to Dr. Phil solve somebody else's issues.

High-Intensity vs. Low-Intensity Workouts

If you need any convincing about why intensity is key to reshaping your body, check out this chart. It shows the results of fifteen weeks of high-intensity exercise (HIE) versus steady-state exercise (SSE) and a control group that did no workout (CONT). The left side shows the overall loss of fat: those who did high-intensity workouts lost an average of 2.5 kilograms (about 5.5 pounds) of pure fat overall and about 3 pounds of belly fat. Those who did steady-state workouts actually gained a little bit of fat. Remember: Weight loss is not fat loss. Steady-state workouts make you "skinny fat."

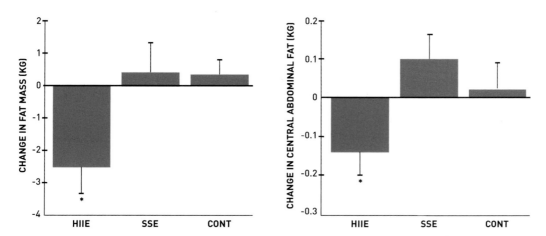

Source: Trapp EG, Chisholm DJ, Freund J, Boutcher SH. "The effects of high-intensity intermittent exercise training on fat loss and fasting insulin levels of young women." *International Journal of Obesity.* 2008;32(4):684–691.

What Happens to Our Bodies When We Don't Exercise

Let's say you'd love to get in shape, just not right now. Like, maybe tomorrow. Or maybe in a few weeks. What's the difference?

The damage we do to our bodies when we don't exercise is substantial. Remember, we evolved to always be moving; this idea of sitting in a chair googling exes is a pretty new invention. Throughout human history, we've been hauling water, hunting game, gathering berries, fighting off saber-toothed tigers, and the like. Primitive man didn't have Seamless.

But when you don't exercise—when you expose your body to the (historically) unusual effects of sitting around, at work and at home—it begins to break down, and quickly. In fact, look at what will happen to you over the next five weeks if you don't exercise:

WEEK ONE: Your diabetes risk rises and your metabolism slows down. In fact, it takes just five days without exercise for your risk to increase, according to University of Missouri researchers. In one study, men were asked to remain more sedentary than usual, and reduced the number of steps they took from about 6,200 to about 1,400. Within one week their glucose tolerance had fallen to 53 percent below normal. Exercise helps prevent diabetes because when we challenge our muscles, it forces them to use sugar stored within our bodies for energy; burning off that sugar improves our ability to manage our overall blood sugar and protects us from diabetes. Once your muscles figure out they don't need to store extra energy, they'll stop drawing sugar out of your bloodstream as effectively.

WEEK TWO: Your muscles begin to waste away, and your fat begins to grow. In fact, even fit people who give up on their workouts for a couple of weeks see dramatic decreases in strength, flexibility, and endurance within about two weeks. A study in the *Journal of Rehabilitative Medicine* found that young men who injured a leg and had it immobilized for two weeks lost between 22 and 34 percent of the muscle mass in that leg. In another study, subjects who reduced their daily activity by about 9,000 steps (or about 4½ miles of walking per day) saw an increase of 7 percent in visceral fat (that's belly fat), and a decrease of more than 2½ pounds of muscle. Meanwhile, the mitochondria in your muscle cells—essentially your cells' "battery packs"—begin to shrink.

Not shrinking: your blood pressure. Your BP readings are generally higher on days that you don't exercise, but within two weeks your arteries begin to adapt to the slower pace of your heart, and your blood pressure ticks up a few points—and stays there, according to a University of Connecticut study in the journal *PLoS.*

WEEK THREE: Your aerobic fitness starts to erode—fast. Aerobic fitness just means the ability of your heart and lungs to deliver oxygen to the rest of your body. In one study, healthy young men who were put on bedrest suffered a 27 percent decrease in aerobic capacity in just twenty days. Meanwhile, your diabetes risk continues to rise: within three weeks of reducing their daily steps, the men in the study I cited earlier saw their glucose tests fall to 79 percent below normal.

WEEK FOUR: You get dumber and more stressed out. A Princeton study found that mice that exercised were better equipped to deal with stress than those that didn't. "Fit" mice exposed to cold water more effectively shut off the anxiety neurons in their brains, while mice that weren't allowed to exercise experienced much greater levels of stress. Some research suggests that when exercise-fueled neurotransmitters are reduced, it can lead to depression and a decrease in cognitive function. As dopamine (your "feel-good" hormone) drops, you feel more anxious and fatigued, making it harder to get back to the gym.

Worse, your blood pressure may now be reset to where it would have been if you hadn't exercised at all.

WEEK FIVE: Your belly is (much) bigger. A study in the *Journal of Strength & Conditioning Research* found that college swimmers who took a five-week exercise break saw their fat mass grow by 12 percent.

Here's the good news: Your muscle cells contain something called myonuclei— basically, the "brains" of the muscle cells. And when you're inactive, muscle cells shrink, but the myonuclei remain intact, according to a study by the National Academy of Sciences. This partly explains why you never forget how to ride a bike once you've mastered the skill: your muscle memory (or muscle "brain") remains intact. For that reason, it's much easier to get back in shape than we imagine. Like flower bulbs sitting in the ground under the snow, our bodies are just waiting to spring forth. We just need to give them a little light and a little heat!

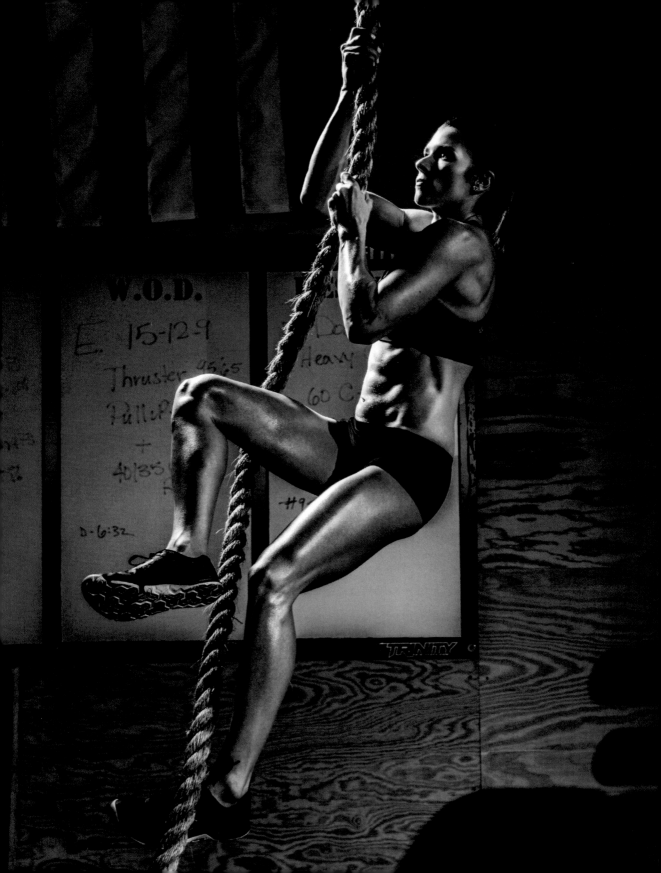

CHAPTER 9

THE CASE FOR WORKING OUT TWICE IN ONE DAY

I know what you're thinking: Who has time to work out two times a day?

Sometimes, we don't, but *sometimes*, we do! I try to do two-a-days whenever I can, because, yes, schedules and work are demanding. And sometimes I find it easier to squeeze in two short workouts (I'm talking twenty minutes, tops) than to set aside time for something longer.

(Shoot, with these short workouts you might even be able to get rid of that gym membership. All they do is take time and money. I love having a home gym—no excuses, and I can cram in a workout so much more easily. And as you'll see, you don't need a lot of space or fancy machines!)

I didn't do two-a-days until the beginning of 2016. I was stuck, and didn't feel like my normal workouts were moving the needle fast enough. Moving to this schedule has been central to taking me to the next level. And if you give it a shot, you'll see it work wonders for you, too.

> "The only easy day was yesterday."
>
> —NAVY SEAL SAYING

Burn More Fat While You Rest!

There are several reasons why two short workouts a day are better than one longer sweat sesh. One of the most compelling is "the afterburn effect."

You've probably heard of the afterburn effect. It refers to the accelerated rate at which your body burns calories—calories it mostly pulls from your fat stores—after you work out. Technically, it's called excess post-exercise oxygen consumption, or EPOC.

After a workout, your body still has a lot of work to do. To return to a resting state, it has to replenish its fuel stores, repair the cells that have been taxed by exercise, rebalance its hormones, and settle down your nervous system. To do that, it breaks down fat stores and burns them using oxygen.

As with a fire, your body can't burn off anything without using oxygen. So researchers measure how many calories we burn by measuring how much oxygen we consume. (The body burns 5 calories to consume 1 liter of oxygen.) It's compelling to think that while you're in the shower or enjoying a post-workout snack, your body is still working hard to help you look your best. In fact, depending on how hard you worked in the gym, your body will burn off an additional 6 to 15 percent more calories after you're done exercising.

The greatest impact on EPOC is that word again: intensity. As intensity increases, so do both the duration and the effectiveness of the afterburn effect. In one study, people who exercised at 75 percent of their maximum continued to burn calories for another 10.5 hours; those who exercised at 50 percent of their max burned calories for only 3.3 hours afterward.

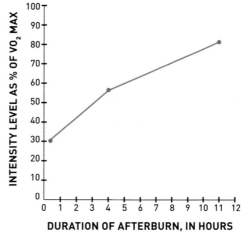

Shorter Workouts, Longer Burn

One of the magic elements of two-a-days, then, is that it gives us not one, but two afterburn opportunities. That means you get more fat burn for the same amount of workout time.

For example, in one study, two groups of men were asked to exercise at a 70 percent intensity for thirty minutes. One group performed the workout for a straight thirty minutes, while the other performed two fifteen-minute workouts, separated by six hours. The researchers measured the subjects post-exercise, and found that the two-a-day group burned about 30 percent more oxygen (i.e., calories) in the forty minutes after their workouts than the single-workout group.

One 30-minute workout
5.3 liters of oxygen = 26.5 calories

Two 15-minute workouts (with 6 hours' rest)
7.4 liters of oxygen = 37 calories

But remember, these subjects were performing the workouts at the same level of intensity. If you crank up just one of those short workouts, you'll see even more gains. And if you crank up both? Unbelievable! When I do two workouts a day, they have to be shorter for me to achieve the level of intensity I want.

That's why an early, intense workout followed by a second workout hours later is a huge double win for team you. The early exercise session keeps your body burning fat at an accelerated rate throughout most of the day, while the later workout just keeps the party going. By exercising before and after work, you could literally plan your day so you're burning extra fat from the moment you wake to the moment you go to sleep . . . and even with your eyes closed!

> "The pain you feel today is the strength you'll feel tomorrow."
>
> —UNKNOWN

How to Build a Two-a-Day Plan

Most of the time, when I can schedule two-a-days, my first workout is an interval cardio workout. I can just run out the door and get it done; it doesn't take me much longer than twenty-five minutes. I do that one first because the one that is most important to me is the HIIT/CrossFit/strength-training workout. So I am totally setting myself up, but in a good way! Then in the afternoon I might even recruit someone to do a WOD (workout of the day in CrossFit slang) with me.

The most common time I do my interval cardio is when I take the dogs out for a run. It dawned on me that I should kill two birds with one stone, and that way all of us can get some good exercise! The workouts are meant to follow the trend of high intensity— I intersperse brief, all-out sprints with a walking recovery. It keeps things moving and keeps it fun! I mean . . . have you ever seen a sprinter without washboard abs?!

I didn't know it at the time, but by doing a strength-training workout and a separate cardio workout, I was actually following the exact protocol that the American Council on Exercise (ACE) recommends for someone who's exercising twice a day.

ACE suggests two-a-day workouts for a few specific purposes. One is for body-sculpting, which involves adding lean muscle and lowering body-fat levels. (That's exactly what we're doing with the *Pretty Intense* program!) The second is for CrossFit-style training, which of course is what the *Pretty Intense* plan most closely resembles.

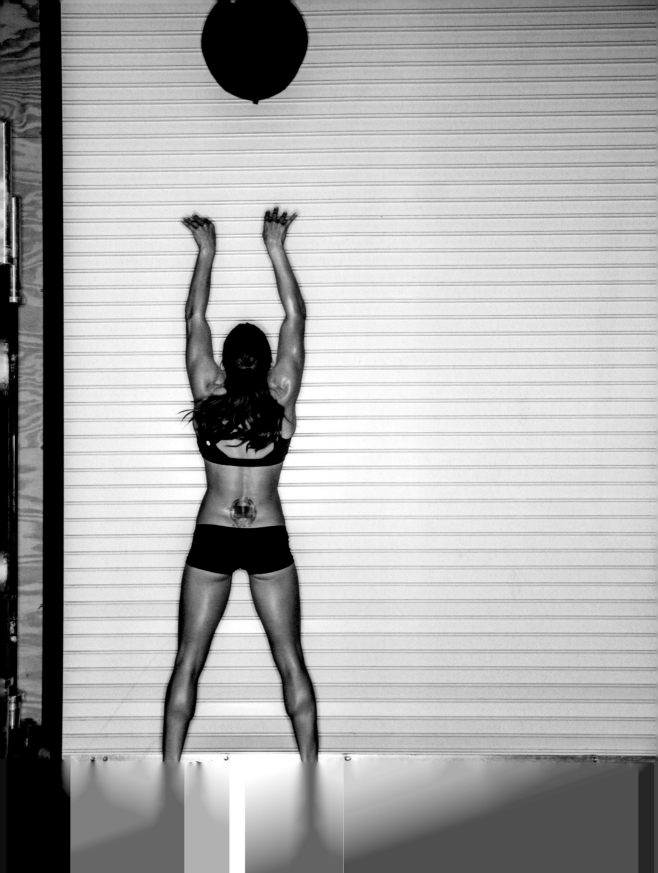

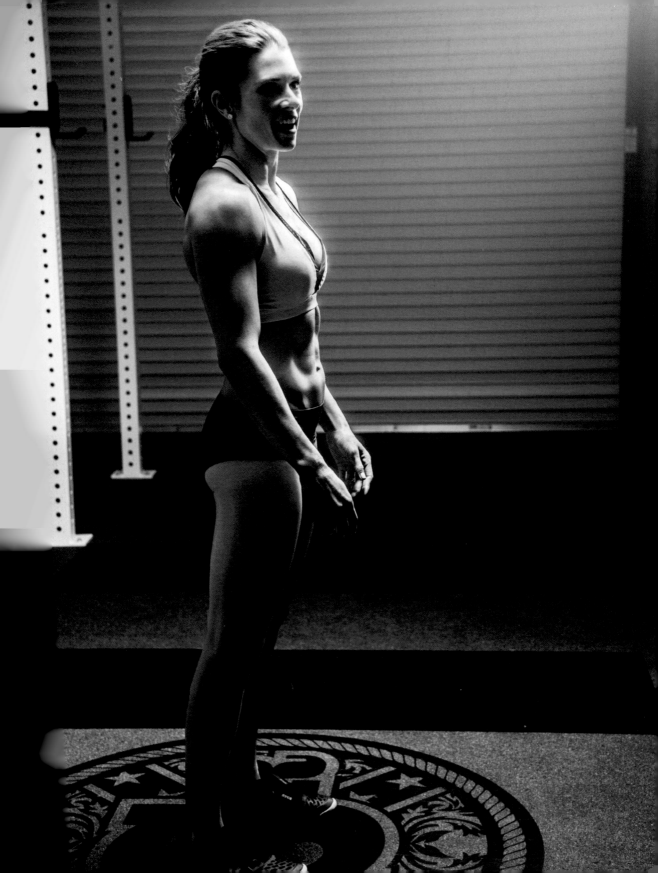

Three things to keep in mind when you're planning a two-a-day schedule:

- Remember my mantra: You can't do two workouts in a day until you've done one!
- Make sure you listen to your body; this level of fitness takes a lot, and if you're injured, you're going to set your progress back.
- Give yourself at least six hours between workouts to allow your body to recover, as well as to take advantage of another huge benefit of two-a-days: the afterburn effect.

Maximum Strength Plan

Let's say you're not sold on the idea of two-a-days, but you'd sure love to work out more. If you can't do two workouts in a day, can you just combine two workouts (say, weight training and cardio) into one big blowout and get the same effect?

No.

I've already explained the unique benefits of exercising twice in one day. At the same time, there are also unique benefits to not doing a single long workout session.

First, combining two workouts back-to-back—say, an intense session with weights followed by a cardio workout—creates what scientists call the "interference effect." Apparently, the body systems that allow us to adapt to intensive weight training (by building strength) and to long, continuous cardio (by building endurance) are at odds with each other; when you try to combine weights-only workouts with long cardio workouts, you render them both less effective than if you did them separately, with sufficient rest in between. (That's why a HIIT program, which builds strength and endurance simultaneously, is so much more effective!)

> "A man's health can be judged by which he takes two at a time—pills or stairs."
>
> —REP. JOAN WELSH

Second, longer workouts just aren't good for your muscles. In fact, training sessions that are longer than forty-five minutes can begin to burn through all the stored energy (called glycogen) in your muscles; once that happens, your body will start looking around for other sources of nourishment. Unfortunately, it's easier and faster to break down muscle tissue than fat tissue, which is why long, slow workouts may help you lose weight, but not fat. (Hence, "skinny fat.") You'll never get the firm, sexy physique you want that way!

On the other hand, shorter, more intense workouts give your muscles time to refuel; the muscles can draw on energy stored elsewhere (i.e., around your waistline) to recharge themselves. In fact, the more muscle you have, the more energy your body burns

The Twice-a-Day Metabolism Trick

How many more calories can you burn by working out twice a day? That depends on how intensely you're working. The more intensity you bring to your exercise—even if those workout sessions are shorter—the greater the boost to your metabolism, and your fat burn.

Consider this: In one study, researchers had a group of trained weight lifters do four sets of eight to twelve reps of eight different exercises. In between, they rested from one to two full minutes, just like a typical weight-training session. A second group did just three sets of three exercises, lifting each weight no more than six times, but they pushed themselves to the max with heavier weights, and rested only twenty seconds in between exercises. As a result, they worked out for only half the time of the first group.

Twenty-two hours later, the group that did the shorter, more intense workouts had a resting metabolism that was 452 calories higher than it was before their workout. The longer, more traditional workout group saw an increase of just 98 calories.

Now, imagine you do an intense workout of that nature twice a day. The difference between your resting calorie burn and that of the average exerciser might look like the chart on the left.

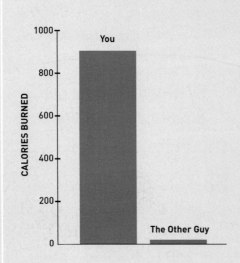

while at rest. According to a study in the *Journal of Clinical Nutrition*, the body uses six calories a day to sustain every pound of muscle, while it uses just two calories a day for each pound of fat. That means the more fat you have, the more fat you'll get; the more muscle you have, the more lean you'll get.

So shorter, two-a-day workouts help build and preserve muscle, leading to more fat burn, and they create a greater afterburn effect, leading to more fat burn. Both of these things are happening when we're not even exercising! That's the fitness equivalent of compound interest.

But there's more.

The Habit That Sticks

While it might seem harder to squeeze in two workouts a day, the facts say otherwise. In one study, researchers prescribed between twenty and forty minutes of exercise, five days a week, to two sets of overweight forty-year-old women. One group was asked to exercise no more than ten minutes at a time, while the other group did their entire workout in one session each day.

You'd think that trying to work out two, three, even four times a day might be discouraging. But in fact, the women who had to exercise more than once a day actually showed up more total days, logged more total exercise time, and lost more weight. *And they saw an improvement in cardiovascular fitness (VO_2 max) that was almost the same as the long-bout exerciser.*

WORKOUT	# DAYS EXERCISED	TOTAL TIME EXERCISED	WEIGHT LOSS	VO_2 MAX INCREASE
2+ PER DAY	87.3	223.8 min	8.9 lbs	5.0%
1 PER DAY	69.1	188.2 min	6.4 lbs	5.6%

In other words, the two-plus workouts per day group squeezed in 15 percent more exercise time and lost 30 percent more weight, even though they weren't allowed to exercise for more than ten minutes at a time!

So whenever you can, keep it short and sweet (and intense). You'll get more benefit from the minutes you put in if you don't put them in all together.

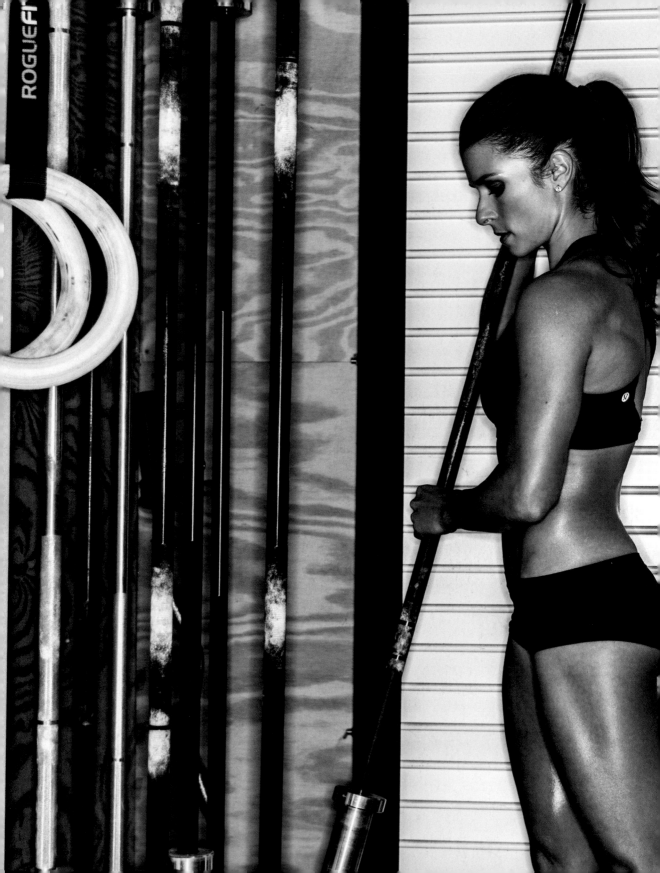

CHAPTER 10

WEIGHTS

Say the words *female weight lifter* and what comes to mind? Probably an unfeminine, thick, overly tanned lady lookin' like a dude.

Guys have no problem jumping into a resistance-training plan. But lifting weights is one of the hardest things to talk women into doing. So many of us buy into the stereotype that a woman who trains with weights will look bulky or less feminine. But that's as far from the truth as can be.

Just take a look around the local gym. You'll see that even the vast majority of men who are lifting weights are having a lot of trouble putting on muscle. In fact, packing on big, bulky muscle is extremely difficult for anybody, but pretty much impossible for women. Unless you're dedicating hours every day in the gym, along with eating a calculated and very protein-heavy diet, you're simply not going to build a hypermuscular physique.

But you will become leaner, firmer, and sexier. Lifting weights helps you drop the weight, but more important, it helps reshape your body to give you a fitter, leaner, and more angular physique. Cardio burns a few more calories during the activity itself, but once you are done, that pretty much ends. When lifting weights, you burn during the workout and for many hours after, resulting in a higher calorie burn overall. Less time + more benefit = no brainer! In fact, if I can accomplish one thing with this book, it's to get you to equate weight-lifting with a very particular female form: mine.

Look at the pictures in this book. Do I look bulky to you? Is there any chance you're going to mistake me for John Cena? No. It's really not something you should worry about. When you start this program, you'll notice parts of your body becoming firmer—not necessarily slimmer, but firmer. That's the first step. As your muscles get stronger, they'll start to demand your fat cells cough it up; within a few weeks, your fat will start to burn away as your body looks for ways to feed your newfound muscle.

"Where the mind goes, the body will follow."

—ARNOLD SCHWARZENEGGER

How I Fixed My Figure

As I said earlier in this book, my workouts used to be long, and slow, and entirely based on "burning calories" so I could get in "great shape." I ran for hours, and I got small. Really small—like 95 pounds. And guess what? I didn't feel, or look, particularly fit. I lacked muscle, and because of that I didn't appear as lean as I truly was because my body was still soft and round instead of sleek and strong.

I honestly thought to myself, *What now?* And the answer was, nothing. There was nothing at the end of that tunnel. Beyond my ability to run really far, I didn't accomplish anything new, or make any new friends, or do anything much to better my body from the inside out.

I had lived in that box for ten years when I found a trainer who recommended I try resistance training. He would send me programs that involved lifting heavy weights at low reps. It was purely a weight-training program, nothing else, so I still continued to run for thirty to forty-five minutes a day. I was surprised to discover how much the weights began to change the way I looked and felt. My body got more angular and looked leaner because I finally had some muscle tone: I wasn't getting bulky or thick, I just looked more fit! Fast-forward to now, and I hardly ever lift less than 65 pounds, and as much as 250 pounds . . . and I weigh probably 20 pounds more in the picture on the bottom. Which one would you pick?

Top photo. Runs for hours and eats very little

Bottom photo. Never does the same workout twice and eats more (very healthy food) than anyone I know!

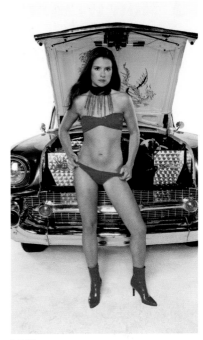

2003

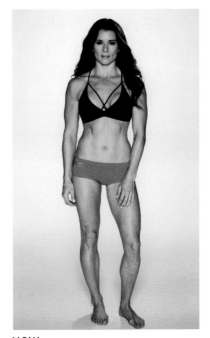

NOW

How Women *Can* Compete with Men

Muscle comes from a number of hormones, but its primary driver is testosterone. The reason men build more muscle than women is simple: Men have, on average, fifteen to twenty times as much testosterone as women. As a result, women only have about half to two-thirds as much muscle as men. That's your natural, hormonal defense against growing "bulky."

And your muscles are nothing to sniff at. Consider this:

- **Women recover from weight training much, much faster than men.** In one study at Ball State University, men who performed bench presses needed forty-eight hours of rest in order to bench press the same amount of weight again, but the women in the study needed just four hours of recovery time.

- **Women's muscles fatigue slower than men's.** Ever notice that when it comes to really hard exercise, men can sorta be babies? Well, in fact, men simply don't have the same level of muscular endurance as women, according to researchers at Marquette University. In any sort of high-intensity workout, an equally fit man will give out before you do.

- **Women's muscles stay stronger with time.** While it may be harder for women to build muscle, studies show that women actually build strength just as efficiently as men do, and suffer less erosion of muscle quality with age.

- **Women's muscles protect them from losing bone density with age.** Our bones lose mineralization more quickly than men's do as we age, but adding muscle is a natural defense against that worry!

Muscle Is Fat's Worst Enemy

Inside your body, muscle and fat are in an endless war. Muscle draws energy away from fat to feed itself, causing the fat to shrink. Fat, in response, sends out hormones called cytokines that increase inflammation and actually work to shrink and weaken muscles, so the fat can claim more turf for itself.

You know which side you want to win. This program is designed to make sure you're on the victorious side.

I've already told you how muscle burns more calories while at rest—three times as much per pound as the same amount of body fat—and how muscle burns away fat to replenish itself after a workout. But lifting weights is also an effective fat-burning workout on its own—much more so than we used to think.

Old-school fitness charts categorize weight-lifting as "moderate" exercise, while running or biking is considered "vigorous." But in 2014, Arizona State researchers using more scientific methods of measuring calorie burn found that weight-training actually burned twice as many calories as previously thought.

And HIIT is the most effective way to burn calories with weights—to reshape your body, melt away fat and replace it with lean, firm, sexy muscle.

Yep, it's that word again: *intensity*. A lot of traditional weight-lifting involves hefting up the weights, then sitting around for a while "recovering." No. I don't have time for that, and neither do you! The *Pretty Intense* HIIT workouts will have you lifting weights while being constantly in motion, moving rapidly from one exercise to the next so you're burning fat as efficiently as possible.

> "Don't ask for a light load; ask for a strong back."
>
> —UNKNOWN

Don't Be Afraid of Heavy

Look around your local Sports Authority. See those little pink and blue weights over there? Those are not for you.

Light weights are useful for physical therapy, but for real exercise, you need real weights. A study in the journal *Medicine & Science in Sports & Exercise* found that women who lifted heavier weights for fewer reps (85 percent of their max load for eight reps) experienced nearly twice as much afterburn effect as those who lifted lighter weights for more repetitions. And remember: Your muscles are just as strong as a man's, and even more resilient. So lift heavy enough that your muscles give out by the eighth

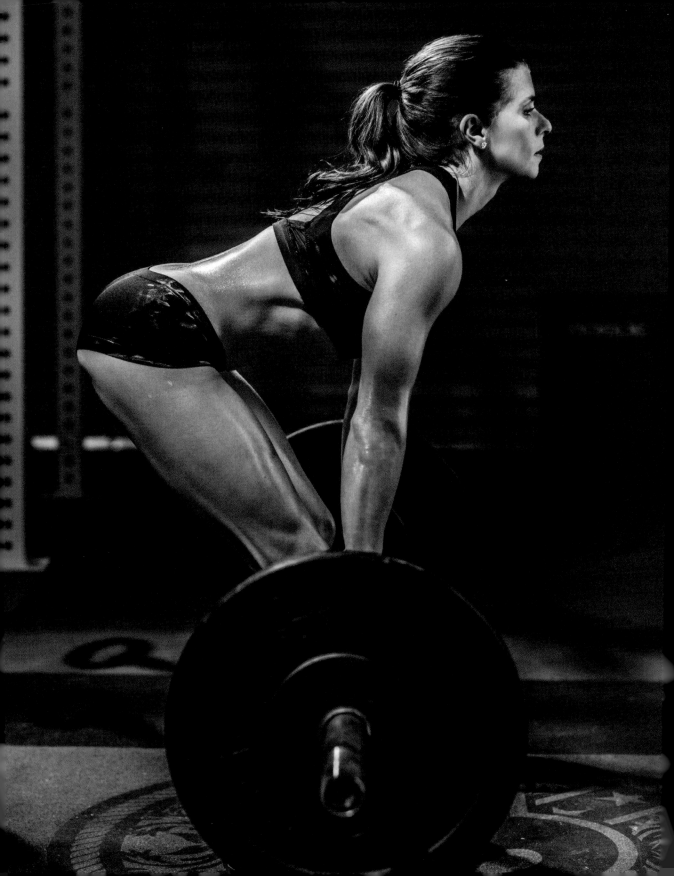

rep, or even earlier; if you can lift a weight twelve or fifteen times, you're spending too much time and not getting enough in return.

The other thing you'll find throughout this program is that I'll ask you to use free weights or your own body weight rather than those fancy machines at the gym. There are two reasons for this: Number one, you'll be able to do my workouts anywhere, so no excuses when you can't get to the gym or you're on vacation. Number two, free weights are simply better for building overall strength. A study at California State University, Chico, compared three types of leg exercises: knee extensions (on a machine), leg presses (also on a machine), and squats (using free weights). The knee-extension group showed a 5 percent increase in strength; the leg-press group showed a 35 percent increase in strength; but the squat group increased their overall strength by 75 percent! Think about that the next time you're tempted to "work out" by sitting down on one of those machines!

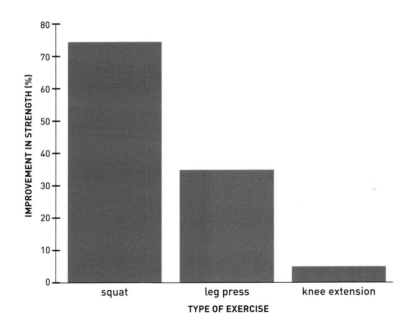

That said, if something hurts, then stop or modify the exercise! Please! Especially if you're feeling pain in joints like your knees, hips, elbows, or shoulders. But, as I said earlier, don't confuse "it hurts" with "it's too hard." That's merely a mental hurdle. These workouts will be over before you know it, so work hard. I respect the fact that your time is valuable; don't waste it resting. Give it your best effort for the short amount of time you have to not only look better but *feel* better, too!

Why We Need to Mix It Up

Ever heard the word *plateau*? In any kind of fitness program, it refers to a sticking point, a point at which, after seeing terrific progress, you suddenly get stuck. You're not getting any stronger, you're not seeing any change in your body. You keep doing what's been working for you, and suddenly it stops working.

Studies show that within six weeks, our muscles adapt to whatever new stimulus we're giving them; while we may see dramatic and highly motivating improvements in strength and endurance over just the first few workouts, eventually that rate of improvement starts to slow. It's why most traditional fitness programs—running, standard weight training, or just about anything—can have their moments of frustration.

There are a number of ways to bust through a plateau: taking time off from one form of exercise to try another; ensuring you're getting enough sleep; exercising your muscles in new and different ways. But the absolute best way to break through a plateau is to not reach one in the first place.

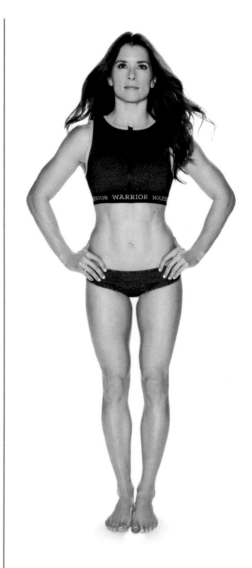

25% Weight Lifter
+
50% CrossFitter
+
20% Sprinter
+
5% Distance Runner
=
PRETTY INTENSE

The *Pretty Intense* Workout plan will never have you doing the same workout twice. My program keeps our muscles challenged all the time, with new exercises, new angles, new approaches. You'll keep getting stronger, and you'll see your endurance and fitness build and build.

One plateau you might see is in weight loss, but like I've said, don't let the numbers on the scale be your guide. Muscle weighs more than fat, so as you're burning away fat and adding muscle, you're not going to see a dramatic drop in pounds—at least not at first. Once you've built that new muscle, it will keep eating away at your fat stores for as long as you keep exercising it, meaning that weight loss will continue for as long as you need it.

You are going to accomplish amazing things with this program. You're going to see changes in your body—in its strength, its endurance, and its overall fitness—that will astound and inspire you. My program is not designed to give you the body of a weight lifter, or a CrossFitter, or a cross-trainer, or a sprinter . . . You are going to work toward a beautiful hybrid of them all. You will lean out and gain muscle. Oh, and you are going to have fun in the process! Seriously!

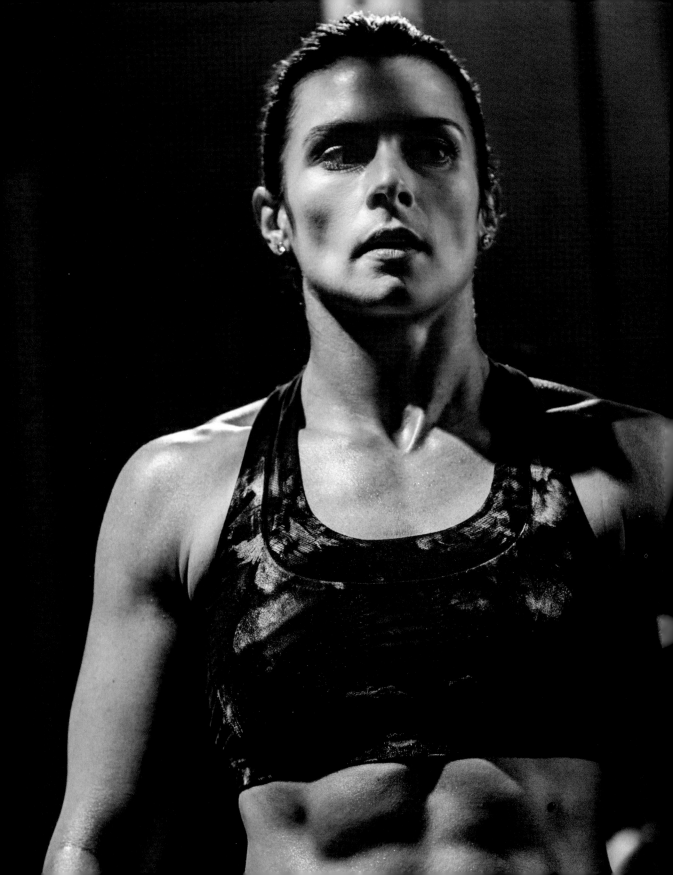

CHAPTER 11

THE *PRETTY INTENSE* WORKOUTS

Twelve weeks.

It's not much time, when you think about it. Call it three months, call it ninety days, call it 2,160 hours. No matter how you parse it, completely changing the way your body looks, feels, and moves in just twelve weeks is going to take work. It's going to take dedication. And most of all, it's going to take intensity.

I've spent the past year pushing my body to the limit, testing out workouts, tweaking and improving, adapting my own exercise regimen into a plan that's perfectly suited for anyone. Yes, it's challenging, but I have proof that it works no matter what your experience or current fitness level is. That proof comes in the form of the hundreds of men and women of all ages and sizes who took

> "You have been criticizing yourself for years, and it hasn't worked. Try approving of yourself and see what happens."
>
> **—LOUISE L. HAY**

part in my test panel—people just like you who dropped pounds while sculpting their bodies and boosting their overall physical and mental health. The *Pretty Intense* Workouts are right for everyone, because they let you use your own body weight for most of the exercises, and they're designed to help you improve your time and performance week after week, proving to yourself that you're getting stronger, fitter, and healthier.

Each week, you'll do seven workouts:

- 3—interval cardio sessions
- 1—upper body workout
- 1—lower body workout
- 1—abs workout
- 1—long circuit

Each workout is designed to take somewhere between twenty and twenty-five minutes, except for the "long circuit," which will take between thirty and forty-five minutes.

Exercise demonstrations

If any of the exercises in this chapter seem unfamiliar to you, or if you just want a primer on form, you can go to PrettyIntense.com to watch a video of me performing each of the moves featured in this book.

Equipment needed

- Chair/bench
- Jump rope
- Slam ball
- Mat

- Tabata timer
- Set of dumbbells (10 pounds)
- Optional—additional dumbbells (5 and 15 pounds)

As you read earlier in the book, doing two workouts a day just a couple of days a week will have a dramatic impact on your overall fitness gains. I realize that we are often slaves to the scheduling demands of others, but thanks to the shortness of these workouts, hopefully you'll be able to squeeze two in a few days a week. (Leave at least six hours between workouts to maximize your gains.) Again, an ideal schedule would look like this:

MON	TUES	WED	THURS	FRI	SAT	SUN
cardio (A.M.) upper body (P.M.)	lower body (A.M. OR P.M.)	cardio (A.M.) abs (P.M.)	cardio (A.M. OR P.M.)	off	long circuit (A.M. OR P.M.)	off

This is just how I would do it, and following this regimen has provided me with maximum strength to perform each workout to the highest of my ability. But the most important thing isn't the schedule you choose. What matters is that you squeeze all seven workouts into your week—and that you perform these workouts with *intensity*.

Here are some terms to familiarize yourself with before you start:

AMRAP: As Many Reps as Possible. If you see AMRAP, it means I've given you a time period in which to do as many repetitions of the exercise as you can.

Ladder: A ladder is when you perform two or more exercises back to back, increasing or decreasing the number of repetitions for each set. For example:

Descending/ascending ladder 15 > 1 > 15
Broad jumps
Air squats

In this case, you'll do fifteen broad jumps followed by fifteen air squats. Then you'll do fourteen broad jumps followed by fourteen air squats, and so on all the way down to one of each. Then you'll start climbing back up the ladder until you're back to fifteen of each exercise.

Rounds: When you see a number of rounds followed by a series of exercises, it means you'll perform each exercise for the prescribed number of repetitions, then move on to the next exercise, then the next. Once you've completed one set of each exercise, that's one complete round. So, for example:

5 ROUNDS:
- 20 knee push-ups
- 20 bent-leg triceps dips
- 20 Supermans
- 20 jumping jacks

In this instance, you'd do twenty of the first exercise, followed by twenty of the next, and so on. Once you've completed twenty of each, that's one round. Start again, and keep going until you've nailed five rounds. You can do this!

Tabata: Tabata training is a type of workout named for Dr. Izumi Tabata, a Japanese researcher who found that four-minute exercises seemed to be optimal for building lean muscle. Ahh, just four minutes!

But those four minutes are intense. For each exercise, you'll:

- Push yourself as hard as you can for 20 seconds.
- Rest for 10 seconds.
- Complete 8 rounds (for a total of 4 minutes).

You'll need a Tabata timer app for your phone to perform this workout, but there are plenty of free options available.

What do you think? Can you handle it?

I know you can.

Get ready. Get set.

Go!

Get Up Off Your Ass!

You've heard of hormones like testosterone and HGH, and how they help us burn fat, right? Well, there's another set of hormones worth learning about: They're called myokines, and researchers didn't even know about them until about 2008. But once you know about them, you're going to want to stand up and pay attention. Seriously.

Myokines are hormones produced by skeletal muscle; when our muscles contract, these hormones are secreted into the bloodstream, where they have all sorts of beneficial effects: They burn fat—both visceral fat (the stuff deep in your belly) and subcutaneous fat (the stuff on your hips and thighs). They improve blood flow and help prevent heart disease. They give your immune system a boost, improve your digestion, and may even help prevent cancer.

The mightiest source of myokines? You're sitting on it. Our legs and backside contain some of the largest muscles in our body, and what have we learned? Muscle burns fat! Throughout human history, they've been constantly contracting to help us stand, walk, run, and jump—and shooting out these stay-young hormones. Problem is, nowadays most of our time is spent sitting on our asses, robbing us of one of our very best weapons for fighting weight gain, disease, and the effects of aging. The more time you spend on your feet, the more time you spend with these muscles contracted—and hence, the more time you spend shooting out myokines. So if you're working a sit-down job, get up and walk around several times each hour. When you're in the gym, make sure you're really focusing on contracting your butt when you're working your lower body. Get your buns working, and work off the rolls!

Week #1 Workout

Cardio		COMPLETED
Cardio 1		
Warm-up:	fast walk 5 min	
20 min:	jog 1 min	☐
	walk 1 min	
Cardio 2		
Warm-up:	fast walk 5 min	
20 min:	10 air squats	
	10 walking lunges (5 each side)	☐
	jog 30 sec	
	walk 1 min	
Cardio 3		
Warm-up:	fast walk 5 min	
For 20 min:	jog 1 min	☐
	walk 30 sec	

Upper Body		COMPLETED
100 butt kickers		
100 jump rope		
100 jumping jacks		
Rest 1 min		
5 rounds:	20 knee push-ups	☐
	20 bent-leg triceps dips	
	20 Supermans	
	20 jumping jacks	

Lower Body		COMPLETED
10 min AMRAP:	20 lunges (10 each side)	
	20 air squats	
	20 step-ups (10 each side)	☐
	20 sumo squat touches	
Rest 2 min		
Repeat		

Abs		COMPLETED
5 min AMRAP:	40 high knees (20 each side)	
	15 feet-anchored sit-ups	
	40 butt kickers (20 each side)	
	15 L-sit toe touches	
Rest 1 min		
5 min AMRAP:	30 ab bikes (15 each side)	☐
	30 ankle touches (15 each side)	
	15 snap jumps	
	30 easy mountain climbers (15 each side)	
Rest 1 min		
Repeat		

Long Circuit		COMPLETED
3 rounds:	10 air squats	
	10 incline push-ups	
	10 planks to downward dog	
Rest 1 min		
Run 8 min		
Rest 2 min		☐
10 min AMRAP:	10 no-push-up burpees	
	20 step-ups (10 each side)	
	30 in/outs	
Rest 2 min		
100 knee push-ups		

Week #2 Workout

Cardio		COMPLETED
Cardio 1		
Warm-up:	fast walk 5 min	
20 min:	jog 2 min	☐
	walk 1 min	
Cardio 2		
Warm-up:	fast walk 5 min	
20 min:	20 air squats	☐
	jog 30 sec	
	walk 1 min	
Cardio 3		
Warm-up:	fast walk 5 min	
20 min:	20 walking lunges (10 each side)	☐
	walk 30 sec	
	jog 30 sec	
	walk 30 sec	

Upper Body		COMPLETED
9 min AMRAP:	5 inchworms	
	10 no push-up burpees	
	15 knee push-ups	
Rest 2 min		
9 min AMRAP:	5 dumbbell thrusters	☐
	10 Supermans	
	15 bent-leg triceps dips	
Rest 1 min		
4 min (20 sec on/20 sec off): plank		

Lower Body	COMPLETED
descending/ascending ladder: 15 > 1 > 15	
broad jumps	☐
air squats	

Abs	COMPLETED
4 rounds: 20 feet-anchored sit-ups	
20 no-push-up burpees	
20 L-sit toe touches	☐
20 straight-leg raises	
30 sec plank	

Long Circuit	COMPLETED
3 rounds: butt kickers 30 sec	
jumping jacks 30 sec	
lunges 30 sec	
rest 30 sec	
Rest 2 min	
400m run (.25 miles)	
30 push-ups	
400m run	
30 feet-anchored sit-ups	
400m run	☐
30 bench jumps	
400m run	
30 commandos (15 each side)	
400m run	
30 straight-leg raises	
400m run	
30 air squats with arms overhead	

Week #3 Workout

Cardio	COMPLETED
Cardio 1	
Warm-up: fast walk 5 min	
20 min: right-side shuffle 20 sec	☐
left-side shuffle 20 sec	
jog 20 sec	
walk 1 min	
Cardio 2	
Warm-up: fast walk 5 min	
15 min: skip 30 sec	☐
walk 30 sec	
Cardio 3	
Warm-up: fast walk 5 min	
20 min: jog 30 sec	☐
walk 30 sec	

Upper Body	COMPLETED
1 min squat jacks	
1 min commandos	
1 min side-to-side quick steps	
1 min knee push-ups	
Rest 1 min	
Repeat the same moves for 30 sec each as fast as you can	
Rest 1 min	☐
1 min no push-up burpees	
1 min bent-leg triceps dips	
1 min jumping jacks	
1 min inchworm and push-up	
Rest 1 min	
Repeat the same moves for 30 sec each as fast as you can	

Lower Body		COMPLETED
5 rounds:	hop overs 40 sec	
	rest 20 sec	
	lunges 40 sec	
	rest 20 sec	
	squat jumps 40 sec	☐
	rest 20 sec	
	alternating squat and kick 40 sec	
	rest 20 sec	

Abs		COMPLETED
5 min AMRAP:	20 right-side plank hip dips	
	20 left-side plank hip dips	
	high knees 30 sec	
Rest 1 min		
5 min AMRAP:	30 mason twists (15 each side)	☐
	30 crossover toe touches (15 each side)	
	20 feet-anchored sit-ups	
Rest 1 min		
Repeat		

Long Circuit		COMPLETED
50 air squats		
Rest 2 min		
21-15-9:	dumbbell swings	
	bench jumps	
	squat jumps	
	dumbbell squat curls and presses	
Rest 2 min		
50 no-push-up burpees		☐
Rest 2 min		
21-15-9:	push-ups	
	butterfly sit-ups	
	shoulder presses	
	curls and presses	

Week #4 Workout

Cardio		COMPLETED
Cardio 1		
Warm-up:	fast walk 5 min	
20 min:	10 no-push-up burpees	☐
	jog 30 sec	
	walk 1 min	
Cardio 2		
Warm-up:	fast walk 5 min	
15 min:	10 broad jumps	☐
	walk 30 sec	
Cardio 3		
Warm-up:	fast walk 5 min	
20 min:	20 hop overs (10 each side)	☐
	jog 30 sec	
	walk 1 min	

Upper Body		COMPLETED
8 rounds:	8 no-push-up burpees	
	8 inchworms	
	8 knee push-ups with elbows in	☐
	8 bent-leg triceps dips	

Lower Body		COMPLETED
3 rounds:	30 air squats	
	30 step-ups (15 each side)	
	30 reverse lunges and knee lifts	
1 min bench toe taps		☐
Rest 1 min		
Repeat		

Abs		COMPLETED
Tabata: Complete the full 4 minute Tabata cycle for each move, then a 1 min rest period before you start the next move.		
	butterfly sit-ups	
	plank	☐
	ab bikes	
	easy mountain climbers	

Long Circuit		COMPLETED
Tabata: Complete the full 4 minute Tabata cycle for each move, then a 1 min rest period before you start the next move.		
	air squats	
	jumping jacks	
	hollow body hold	
2 rounds:	100 hop overs	
	50 lunges (25 each side)	
	100 jump ropes	☐
	50 slam balls	
Rest 2 min		
3 rounds:	10 curls and presses	
	10 reverse flies	
	10 lateral raises	

Week #5 Workout

Cardio		COMPLETED
Cardio 1		
Warm-up:	walk 2 min	
	jog 2 min	
	walk 1 min	☐
20 min:	run 30 sec	
	walk 1 min	
Cardio 2		
Warm-up:	walk 2 min	
	jog 2 min	
	walk 1 min	☐
20 min:	run 3 min	
	walk 2 min	
Cardio 3		
Warm-up:	walk 2 min	
	jog 2 min	
	walk 1 min	☐
20 min:	20 walking lunges (10 each side)	
	run 20 sec	
	walk 1 min	

Upper Body		COMPLETED
50-40-30-20-10	slam balls	
	straight-leg triceps dips	☐
	commandos	

Lower Body

		COMPLETED
9 min AMRAP:	20 jumping lunges (10 each side)	
	20 weighted sumo squats	
	20 step-ups and knee lifts	
	10 squat jumps	
Rest 1 min		
9 min AMRAP:	10 broad jumps	☐
	20 step-ups (10 each side)	
	20 weighted lunges (10 each side)	
	10 tuck jumps	
5 min:	wall sit and arms overhead 30 sec	
	rest 30 sec	

Abs

		COMPLETED
8 min AMRAP:	30 hip dips (15 each side)	
	20 no-push-up burpees	
	10 hollow rocks	
Rest 1 min		
8 min:	30 ab bikes (15 each side)	☐
	20 mason twists (10 each side)	
	10 straight-leg raises and hip lifts	
Rest 1 min		
Tabata: full mountain climbers		

Long Circuit

	COMPLETED
800m run (.5 miles)	
50 bench jumps	
50 push-ups	
Rest 3 min	
800m run	
50 in/outs and snap jump	
50 dumbbell thrusters	☐
Rest 3 min	
800m run	
50 full mountain climbers (25 each side)	
50 full burpees	

Week #6 Workout

Cardio		COMPLETED
Cardio 1		
Warm-up:	jog 3 min	
	walk 2 min	
20 min:	10 no-push-up burpees and jumps	☐
	run 30 sec	
	walk 1 min	
Cardio 2		
Warm-up:	jog 3 min	
	walk 2 min	☐
15 min:	run 30 sec	
	walk 30 sec	
Cardio 3		
22 min:	walk 1 min	
	skip 1 min	☐
	run 1 min	

Upper Body		COMPLETED
4 rounds:	20 full burpees	
	20 commandos (10 each side)	
	20 dumbbell thrusters	☐
	20 push-ups with elbows in	

Lower Body	COMPLETED
Tabata: Rest 1 min between each movement	
air squats	
hop overs	☐
in/out squat jumps	
jump ropes	

Abs	COMPLETED
50 jump rope	
50 full mountain climbers (25 each side)	
50 jump rope	
50 mason twists (25 each side)	
50 jump ropes	
50 butterfly sit-ups	
50 jump ropes	☐
50 seated in/outs	
50 jump ropes	
50 snap jumps	
50 jump ropes	
50 hip dips (25 each side)	
Repeat	

Long Circuit		COMPLETED
50-40-30-20-10	weighted overhead lunges	
	air squats	
	bent-knee sit-ups	
Rest 3 min		
3 rounds:	30 hop overs (15 each side)	☐
	15 burpees and tuck jumps	
	rest 1 min	
Tabata: push-ups		

Week #7 Workout

Cardio		COMPLETED
Cardio 1		
Warm-up:	jog 4 min	
	walk 1 min	
20 min:	10 butt kickers	☐
	10 high knees	
	run 30 sec	
	walk 1 min	
Cardio 2		
20 min:	walking lunge 30 sec	
	walk 30 sec	☐
	run 1 min	
	walk 30 sec	
Cardio 3		
Warm-up:	jog 4 min	
	walk 1 min	☐
20 min:	run 30 sec	
	walk 1 min	

Upper Body		COMPLETED
3 rounds:	downward dog 30 sec	
	5 reverse tabletop swings	
	3 wall walks	
Rest 1 min		
100 jump ropes / 5 Superman push-ups		
80 jump ropes / 10 Superman push-ups		
60 jump ropes / 15 Superman push-ups		
40 jump ropes / 20 Superman push-ups		
20 jump ropes / 25 Superman push-ups		☐
40 jump ropes / 20 Superman push-ups		
60 jump ropes / 15 Superman push-ups		
80 jump ropes / 10 Superman push-ups		
100 jump ropes / 5 Superman push-ups		
Rest 1 min		
Tabata: push-ups		

Lower Body	COMPLETED
10 tuck jumps	
20 squat jumps	
30 jumping lunges (15 each side)	
40 step-ups (20 each side)	
50 air squats	
40 step-ups (20 each side)	☐
30 jumping lunges (15 each side)	
20 squat jumps	
10 tuck jumps	
Rest 3 min	
2 rounds: 50 weighted sumo squats	
50 weighted lunges (25 each side)	

Abs	COMPLETED
6 rounds: 10 V-ups	
20 planks knee to elbow (10 each side)	
10 hollow rocks	☐
20 twisting sit-ups with feet elevated (10 each side)	
rest 1 min	

Long Circuit	COMPLETED
Run 10 min	
Rest 3 min	
25 slam balls / 25 push-ups	
20 slam balls / 20 push-ups	
15 slam balls / 15 push-ups	
10 slam balls / 10 push-ups	
5 slam balls / 5 push-ups	
Rest 3 min	
50 ab bikes (25 each side) / 50 full mountain climbers (25 each side)	
40 ab bikes / 40 full mountain climbers	
30 ab bikes / 30 full mountain climbers	☐
20 ab bikes / 20 full mountain climbers	
10 ab bikes / 10 full mountain climbers	
Rest 3 min	
25 tuck jumps / 25 squat jumps	
20 tuck jumps / 20 squat jumps	
15 tuck jumps / 15 squat jumps	
10 tuck jumps / 10 squat jumps	
5 tuck jumps / 5 squat jumps	

Week #8 Workout

Cardio		COMPLETED
Cardio 1		
24 min:	run 2 min	☐
	walk 1 min	
Cardio 2		
Warm-up:	jog 4 min	
	walk 1 min	☐
20 min:	10 squat jumps	
	run 30 sec	
	walk 1 min	
Cardio 3		
Warm-up:	jog 4 min	
	walk 1 min	☐
15 min:	sprint 30 sec	
	walk 30 sec	

Upper Body		COMPLETED
6 min AMRAP:	15 dumbbell squat curls and presses	
	30 plank shoulder taps (15 each side)	
	16 dumbbell press (8 each side)	
	8 inchworm + push-up with elbows in	
Rest 1 min		
6 min AMRAP:	15 decline push-ups	☐
	15 full burpees	
	15 reverse flies	
	15 slam balls	
Rest 1 min		
Repeat		

Lower Body	COMPLETED
Butt kickers + arms up 1 min	
Yogi squat 30 sec	
Jumping jacks 1 min	☐
Yogi squat 30 sec	
High knees 1 min	

Lower Body (continued)		COMPLETED
Yogi squat 30 sec		
Repeat		
15 min AMRAP:	10 full burpees	☐
	10 reverse lunge + knee hop (5 each side)	
	10 sumo squat jumps with 2 sec hold at the bottom	

Abs		COMPLETED
6 min AMRAP:	15 roll back to stand	
	15 plank in/outs + snap jumps	
	15 tuck jumps	
Rest 1 min		
6 min AMRAP:	15 right-side sit-ups	☐
	15 left-side sit-ups	
	15 straight-leg raise + hip lift	
Rest 1 min		
Repeat		

Long Circuit	COMPLETED
100 jump ropes	
90 air squats	
80 lunges (40 each side)	
70 butterfly sit-ups	
60 push-ups with elbows in	
50 step-ups (25 each side)	
40 mason twists (20 each side)	
30 dumbbell push press	
20 burpees	
10 broad jumps	☐
20 burpees	
30 dumbbell push presses	
40 mason twists (20 each side)	
50 step-ups (25 each side)	
60 push-ups with elbows in	
70 butterfly sit-ups	
80 lunges (40 each side)	
90 air squats	
100 jump ropes	

Week #9 Workout

Cardio		COMPLETED
Cardio 1		
24 min:	right-side shuffle 30 sec	
	left-side shuffle 30 sec	☐
	walk 1 min	
	sprint 30 sec	
	walk 30 sec	
Cardio 2		
Warm-up:	jog 4 min	
	walk 1 min	
20 min:	10 jumping lunges	☐
	15 air squats	
	sprint 20 sec	
	walk 1 min	
Cardio 3		
Warm-up:	jog 4 min	
	walk 1 min	
15 min:	run 20 sec	☐
	sprint 10 sec	
	walk 30 sec	

Upper Body		COMPLETED
3 rounds:	100 jump rope	
	3 wall walks	
Rest 2 min		☐
15 min AMRAP:	10 man makers	
	20 dumbbell swings	
	handstand hold 30 sec	

Lower Body		
Tabata: Rest 1 min after each move		
	jump ropes	
	squat jumps	
	jumping lunges	
10 min AMRAP:	30 side sumo squats + kicks (15 each side)	☐
	30 weighted step-ups	
	20 broad jumps	
	20 weighted reverse lunges (10 each side)	

Abs

		COMPLETED
3 rounds:	twisting sit-ups with feet elevated 1 min	
	rest 30 sec	
	upright ab bikes 1 min	
	rest 30 sec	
	hip dips 1 min	
	rest 30 sec	☐
	double mountain climbers 1 min	
	rest 30 sec	
	high knees 1 min	
	rest 30 sec	

Long Circuit

	COMPLETED
Jumping lunges 1 min	
Air squats 1 min	
Squat jumps 1 min	
Alternating side-step sumo squats 1 min	
No-push-up burpees 1 min	
Lunges 1 min	
Repeat the same moves for 30 sec each as fast as you can	
Rest 3 min	
Ab bikes 1 min	
Full mountain climbers 1 min	
Butterfly sit-ups 1 min	
L-sit toe touches 1 min	☐
Hip dips 1 min	
Crossover toe touches 1 min	
Repeat each move for 30 sec each as fast as you can	
Rest 3 min	
Push-ups 1 min	
Bent-leg triceps dips 1 min	
Plank in/outs 1 min	
Full burpees 1 min	
Snap jumps 1 min	
Commandos 1 min	
Repeat each move for 30 sec each as fast as you can	

Week #10 Workout

Cardio		COMPLETED
Cardio 1		
20 min:	walk 45 sec	
	run 30 sec	☐
	sprint 15 sec	
Cardio 2		
Warm-up:	jog 4 min	
	walk 1 min	☐
20 min:	sprint 30 sec	
	walk 30 sec	
Cardio 3		
Warm-up:	jog 4 min	
	walk 1 min	
20 min:	20 hop overs (10 each side)	☐
	run 30 sec	
	walk 30 sec	

Upper Body		COMPLETED
Tabata: Rest 1 min between movements		
	push-ups	
	bent-leg triceps dips	
	jump rope	☐
	slam balls	
	handstand holds	

Lower Body		COMPLETED
10 min AMRAP:	15 burpee hop overs	
	20 double-pulse squat jumps	
	20 dumbbell back squats	
	30 jumping lunges (15 each side)	
Rest 2 min		☐
10 min AMRAP:	15 burpee bench jumps	
	30 reverse lunges + knee hops (15 each side)	
	20 crossover jump squats (10 each side)	
	30 bench hops	

Abs	COMPLETED
10 burpee tuck jumps	
20 V-ups	
30 twisting sit-ups with feet elevated (15 each side)	
40 hip lifts	
50 weighted mason twists (25 each side)	☐
60 butterfly sit-ups	
70 snap jumps	
80 ab bikes (40 each side)	
Plank hold 90 sec	
100 alternating side squats + front kicks (50 each side)	

Long Circuit	COMPLETED
Run 1 mile	
100 sit-ups	
100 push-ups	
100 air squats	☐
100 dumbbell push press	
Run 1 mile	

Week #11 Workout

Cardio		COMPLETED
Cardio 1		
Warm-up:	jog 4 min	
	walk 1 min	☐
20 min:	run 1 min	
	walk 1 min	
Cardio 2		
Warm-up:	jog 4 min	
	walk 1 min	
15 min:	5 tuck jumps	☐
	10 air squats	
	sprint 30 sec	
	walk 30 sec	
Cardio 3		
20 min:	run 4 min	☐
	walk 1 min	

Upper Body		COMPLETED
7 min AMRAP:	20 squat curls and presses	
	20 full burpees	
	20 reverse flies	
Rest 1 min		
7 min AMRAP:	20 slam ball push-ups (10 each side)	☐
	20 lateral raises	
	20 slam balls	
Rest 1 min		
Repeat		

Lower Body

		COMPLETED
5 min AMRAP:	50 jump ropes	
	25 air squats	
Rest 1 min		
50 bench jumps		
50 jumping lunges (25 each side)		
50 hop overs (25 each side)		☐
50 dumbbell thrusters		
50 dumbbell back squats		
50 bench hops (25 each side)		
50 double mountain climbers		

Abs

		COMPLETED
3 rounds:	50 high knees (25 each side)	
	50 full mountain climbers (25 each side)	
	50 butt kickers (25 each side)	
	50 weighted mason twists (25 each side)	
	rest 30 sec	
3 rounds:	20 tuck jumps	☐
	20 twisting sit-ups with feet elevated (10 each side)	
	20 snap jumps	
	20 knee-ups	
	rest 30 sec	

Long Circuit

		COMPLETED
3 rounds:	60 jump ropes	
	60 jumping jacks	
	yogi squat 60 sec	
Rest 1 min		
21-15-9:	dumbbell thrusters	
	full burpees	
Rest 5 min		☐
3 rounds:	30 push-ups with elbows in	
	30 slam balls	
	30 bench jumps	
Rest 2 min		
Tabata: hollow body hold		

Week #12 Workout

Cardio		COMPLETED
Cardio 1		
Warm-up:	jog 4 min	
	walk 1 min	☐
20 min:	run 40 sec	
	walk 20 sec	
Cardio 2		
Warm-up:	jog 4 min	
	walk 1 min	
20 min:	10 jumping lunges (5 each side)	☐
	10 air squats	
	run 30 sec	
	walk 30 sec	
Cardio 3		
Warm-up:	jog 4 min	
	walk 1 min	☐
20 min:	sprint 20 sec	
	walk 40 sec	

Upper Body		COMPLETED
50 jumping jacks		
40 air squats		
30 snap jumps		
20 squat jumps		
10 push-ups		☐
Rest 2 min		
20 min AMRAP:	5/5, 10/10, 15/15, 20/20, 25/25, etc.	
	dumbbell thrusters	
	burpee hop overs	

Lower Body		COMPLETED
6 min AMRAP:	12 bench jumps	
	12 bench knee pulls (12 each side)	☐
	12 step-ups (6 each side)	
Rest 3 min		

Lower Body (continued)		COMPLETED
6 min AMRAP:	12 slam ball sumo squats	
	12 slam ball toe taps (12 each side)	
	12 slam ball hop overs (6 each side)	
Rest 3 min		☐
6 min AMRAP:	12 broad jumps	
	12 dumbbell thrusters	
	12 dumbbell back squats	

Abs		COMPLETED
2 rounds:	20 V-ups	
	20 butterfly sit-ups	
	20 L-sit toe touches	
Tabata: full moutain climbers (25 each side)		
Rest 1 min		
2 rounds:	20 weighted mason twists (10 each side)	
	20 upright ab bikes (10 each side)	☐
	20 crossover toe touches (10 each side)	
Tabata: plank knee to elbow		
Rest 1 min		
2 rounds:	20 right-side sit-ups	
	20 left-side sit-ups	
	20 hip lifts	
Tabata: hollow body hold		

Long Circuit		COMPLETED
8 min AMRAP:	200m run (.12 miles)	
	rest 30 sec	
Rest 4 min		
8 min AMRAP:	12 slam balls	
	12 straight-leg triceps dips	
	12 decline push-ups	
Rest 4 min		
8 min AMRAP:	12 tuck jumps	☐
	12 jumping lunges (6 each side)	
	12 air squats	
Rest 4 min		
8 min AMRAP:	12 plank in/outs + snap jumps	
	12 bent-knee sit-ups	
	12 weighted mason twists (6 each side)	

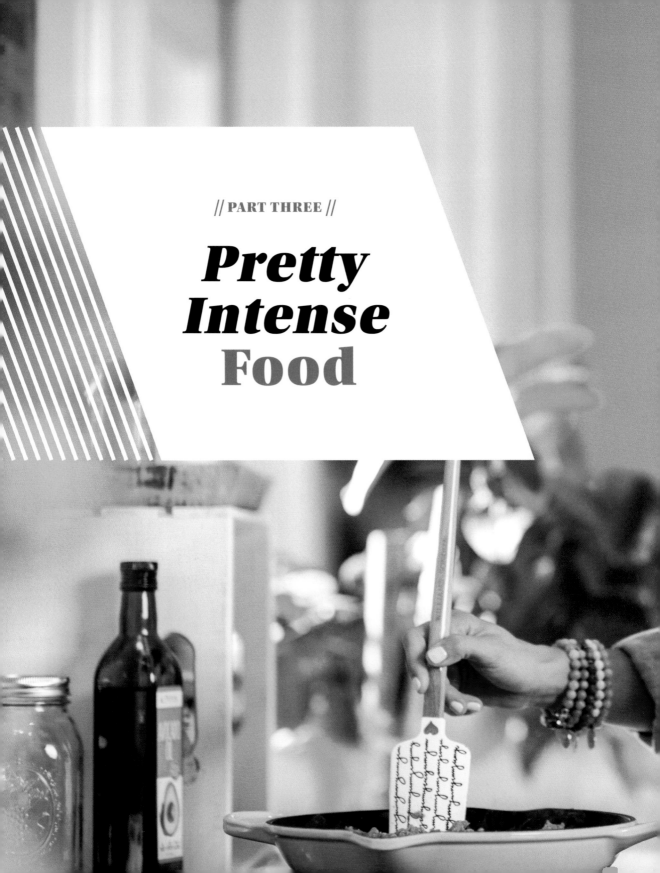

// PART THREE //

Pretty Intense Food

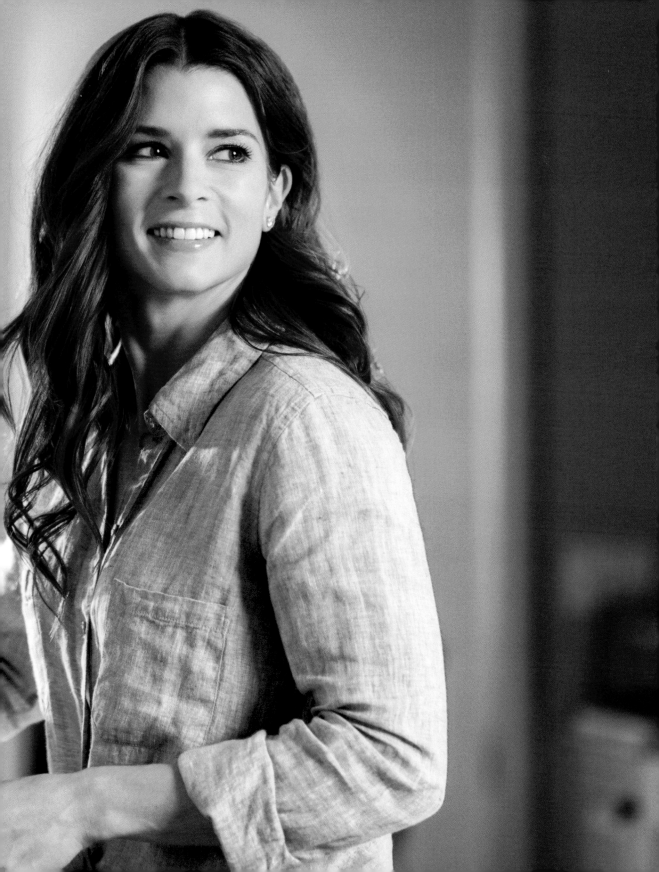

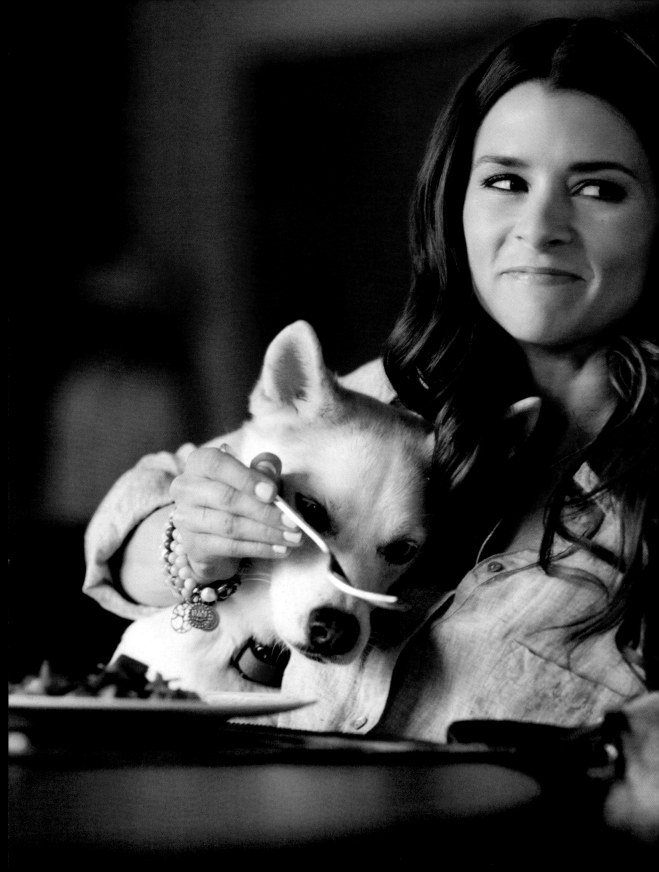

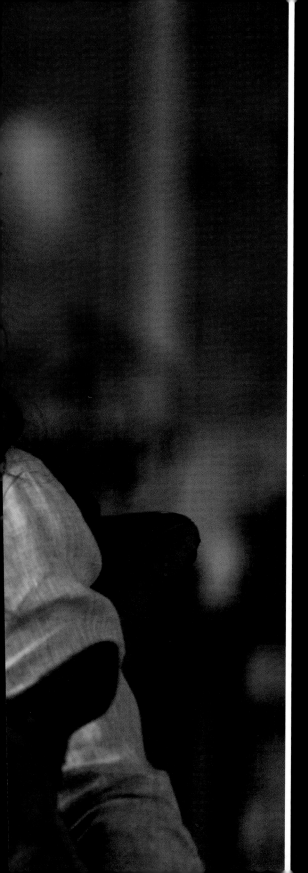

CHAPTER 12

EAT REAL FOOD

How much human hair have you eaten this week?

Chances are, a lot more than you think. If you're like most Americans, you've also eaten plenty of sand, wood pulp, and petroleum products as well.

In fact, if you've consumed a slice of bread, a scoop of ice cream, or a fast-food burger recently, you've almost certainly enjoyed one of these delicacies. They're all common ingredients in packaged foods and restaurant meals.

But they're not real food.

Additives like these are in just about every packaged food we eat, and most of our restaurant meals as well. And by constantly bombarding ourselves with things that aren't food, we're creating a low level of chronic inflammation throughout our bodies. Inflammation plays a major role in weight gain, and puts us at greater risk for heart disease, diabetes, Alzheimer's, and just about every other disease worth freaking out about.

Inflammation is the key to everything. Inflammation is your body's response to foods and additives it deems

> "Don't eat anything your great-grandmother wouldn't recognize as food."
>
> —MICHAEL POLLAN

unhealthy. And perhaps the most significant reason the *Pretty Intense* eating plan has worked so well for me and for my test panel is that it dramatically reduces inflammation and allows your body to return to its natural, healthy state.

Coming Back to Planet Earth

Mother Earth has a lot to offer us from a food perspective. The dirt grows tasty food, the rain waters it, and the sun ripens it. The earth also feeds the animals we consume.

Most of us understand this. We are getting smarter about what we eat and realizing how important it is to feed our bodies with healthy food. But it's not as easy as it seems.

The supermarket is stacked with bags and boxes of edibles that aren't actually real food: stuff that's sold as healthy (foods that claim to be "lite" or "diet" or "enriched"), or stuff labeled "natural" (a word that means nothing when it appears on a food label). We want to do the right thing for ourselves and our families, but it gets harder all the time. That's why it's so important to eat real food and avoid processed foods. A study in the *Journal of the World Public Health Nutrition Association* found that the increase in "ultra-processed" food—food that includes ingredients that aren't, in fact, food—may be *the main cause* for the rise in obesity around the world.

What do you eat that's not food? The next time you go to the supermarket, take a moment to scan the ingredients list on the foods you buy. A good rule of thumb: Anything with more than five ingredients probably contains stuff that's not food. You probably already know that high-fructose corn syrup is a man-made sweetener that many researchers believe is worse for you than sugar, but you might not be on the lookout for some other additives that are in many, many packaged foods. Stuff like BHA (butylated hydroxyanisole, a preservative made from petroleum), sodium nitrate (an antimicrobial substance), silicon dioxide (it's sand!), cellulose (it's wood chips!), L-cysteine (a dough conditioner made most often from human hair), tartrazine (a yellow food dye linked to learning and concentration disorders), and about three thousand other additives that can be legally used to "enhance" our food.

Wood chips, human hair, sand, petroleum—that's not food. Yet we eat so much of these (again, just look at what's in your pantry) that we're actually changing our own bodies.

A 2015 study in the journal *Nature* found that chemical emulsifiers—compounds that give packaged foods like ice cream their smooth consistency—cause an increase in the growth of unhealthy bacteria in our guts. That can lead to the inflammation that causes not only obesity but all those other health issues I mentioned. In fact, about 40 percent of the bacteria species that naturally occur in our bodies have gone extinct over the past sixty years, according to Emeran Mayer, MD, PhD, a brain researcher at UCLA. The proper balance of gut bacteria—what's called your microbiome—is crucial to keeping you slim and healthy.

> "Eat like you give a damn about yourself."
>
> —UNKNOWN

How "Healthy" Is Healthy?

Like I said, it's not easy to figure out the right way to fuel your body. As a teenager, I lived in England for three years, racing Formula cars. Back then I would go to the local bookstore, which also had a coffee shop, and I would order a large latte (which I would not order now) and sit down with a stack of health and fitness books.

I have always been interested in the human body and how it works, and I spent hours flipping through the pages learning new ways to take care of myself. It was the beginning of my experimentation with diets: I think the first phase was low-fat, then low-carb, then dairy-free, then whole grain, then a 40/30/30 balance . . . Then I turned my world upside down with a blood test.

At the beginning of 2013, I took a test that scanned my blood against the ninety-six most common foods. Before I tell you my results, let me tell you generally what I used to eat so you can understand how shocked I was.

BREAKFAST: oatmeal

SNACK: egg whites with goat cheese

LUNCH: whole-grain sandwich with deli meat

SNACK: Greek yogurt with granola and fruit

DINNER: salmon, rice, and veggies

Pretty healthy, right? In fact, except perhaps for the deli meat, the average doctor would say I was eating as healthy as possible.

So, when the test said I had an "extremely high" reaction to egg whites, egg yolks, gluten, yeast, and all dairy items, I wanted to cry! All that discipline had been doing my body no good at all! I began to wonder if the reason I sometimes felt bloated and fatigued had something to do with my reaction to those foods.

That test changed my life. Shortly after I cut those foods out, I realized I had a higher and more consistent energy level day after day. I also did not feel uncomfortable after eating, ever.

Since then I have experimented with a variety of foods, and I've added eggs back into my life simply because I've noticed little if any reaction to them. (And eggs are the most bioavailable source of protein per calorie known to man.) But the *Pretty Intense* plan cuts as much gluten and dairy out of your diet as possible.

(If you ever feel bloated after a meal, it's a sign that your body is reacting to the foods you ate. It's not necessarily a "food allergy," but it may be that your body is react-ing to the foods in a way that can cause inflammation and, eventually, weight gain. Try eliminating wheat from your diet entirely for two weeks and see if you feel better. Then do the same with dairy. You'll be amazed how effective this is—as I'll explain in the fol-lowing paragraphs.)

How My Diet Got *Pretty Intense*

The exact diet plan outlined in this book started at the beginning of 2016. I had gained several pounds of flab after doing a hormone treatment to freeze my eggs. I had never experienced the power of hormones on the body, but I was amazed by how different I looked and felt after undergoing estrogen treatment. I didn't do anything different food-wise, and had to refrain from working out for only two weeks, but I gained *fat* from nowhere! I was super frustrated and decided I needed to do something new and aggressive to get it off.

So in a way, my hormone treatment gave birth to what you're holding in your hands now: *Pretty Intense.*

I began doing two-a-day workouts as often as I could, and after a few weeks of that, I decided to try eating Paleo. I had heard all about Paleo from doing CrossFit (many CrossFit enthusiasts eat this way), but I always had a pretty harsh judgment against it. To me, a traditional Paleo program just didn't offer enough food. But like I said, I needed to try something aggressive!

Paleo is based on the idea that you only eat foods that were available to ancient man before the invention of agriculture. So no grains, no dairy, no beans or legumes, no added sugars or preservatives. Instead, you focus on naturally raised meats, vegetables, fruits, and nuts.

My intention was to only do it for a week or two to reset my body with less sugar and more veggies. Well . . . I felt so good, and saw such amazing results, that I never quit.

It was not that hard to do, and I loved both the change in food and the results I was starting to see. I was starting to actually see upper body muscles and abs! *What?!* Let me tell you, people, I have worked out hard and I have been really picky with food, but these results were by far my best. Paleo formed the origins of *Pretty Intense*, which I've continued to tweak until I created the most effective plan I've ever put myself on. That is why I am writing this book.

The longer I have eaten like this, the more I have thought about it, and it's become clear: It's all about eating real food! Sweet potatoes come from the ground, maple syrup comes out of a tree, carrots grow in the dirt, bees make honey, and hopefully we can all find more and more pasture-raised, grain-free, cruelty-free animals for protein. Because what our animals eat becomes what we eat, too.

I don't see ever getting too far from these principles. Real food is medicine, and I like to put the highest-quality food into the only body I will ever have.

The Trouble with Bread

Of all the changes I made to my diet, giving up bread—as well as pasta, pastries, and other products made with wheat—has made the greatest impact.

Now, you might be thinking, "What's the problem with bread? That's real food, right?" Yes and no. First of all, most commercial breads—even whole-grain breads—have a wild array of ingredients. Here's a sample of what's in one popular whole-wheat bread: high-fructose corn syrup, soybean oil, calcium propionate, datem, soy lecithin. Not food!

One of the things that bread conditioners like datem and L-cysteine do is enhance the strength of gluten, a protein that's found in wheat. That makes the dough light and airy. It's also making a lot of us sick.

You may know someone who is gluten-intolerant, or who has been diagnosed with celiac disease, a serious form of wheat allergy. For someone like this, just a couple of croutons can trigger an immune response that causes inflammation—and eventually real damage—in the small intestine. But you don't need a diagnosis to suffer damage to your digestive tract: a 2011 study found that gluten causes gastrointestinal symptoms in people even if they don't have celiac disease.

In 2013, researchers found that in mouse studies, a gluten-free diet led to reduced body weight, and inflammation and insulin resistance, and a 2016 study linked another protein in wheat, amylase-trypsin inhibitors (ATIs), to inflammation in the lymph nodes, kidneys, spleen, and brain, and suggested that it could be linked to arthritis, asthma, and fatty liver disease, among other things.

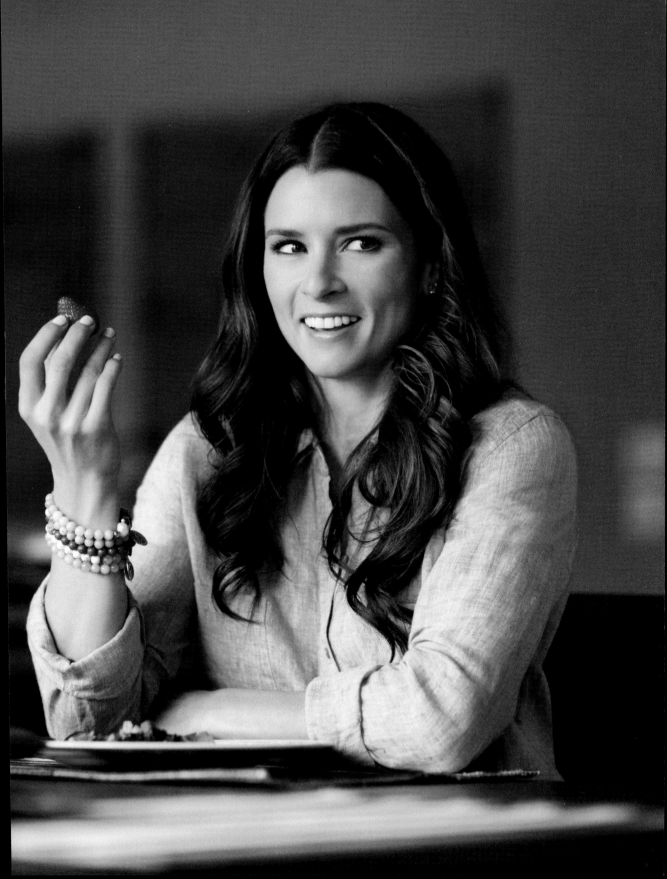

So while you may not follow every piece of dietary advice in this book, the one thing I urge you to do is to give up gluten—at least for a couple of weeks. I'm pretty sure that not eating wheat—and eating real food, not fake food—will make an instant impact on how you look and feel.

How Gluten Makes You Fat

You eat a slice of bread. Your stomach breaks down the bread
into its basic parts—among them, the protein gluten—
and sends it all down to the small intestine.

The immune system in your small intestine identifies the gluten
as a dangerous substance and produces antibodies.

The antibodies attack a digestive enzyme that helps
hold together the lining of your small intestine.

Your small intestine becomes "leaky" as food particles, toxins,
and microbes escape through openings in the lining of your
small intestine and move into your bloodstream and lymph system.

Your immune system goes into overdrive, attacking these toxins
and causing inflammation throughout your body—just as the
fight against a cold virus causes inflammation in your nose.

Inflammation interferes with your body's hormones,
particularly leptin, which controls metabolism and appetite.
You become fatigued as your body enters a low-level "starvation mode,"
automatically burning fewer calories at rest while signaling
your brain to search out more calories from food. Boom: weight gain.

Worksheet: Is It Real Food?

Before you eat your next meal, let's find out whether what you're eating is made up of actual food. Take a look at the ingredients list on each packaged food you're using.

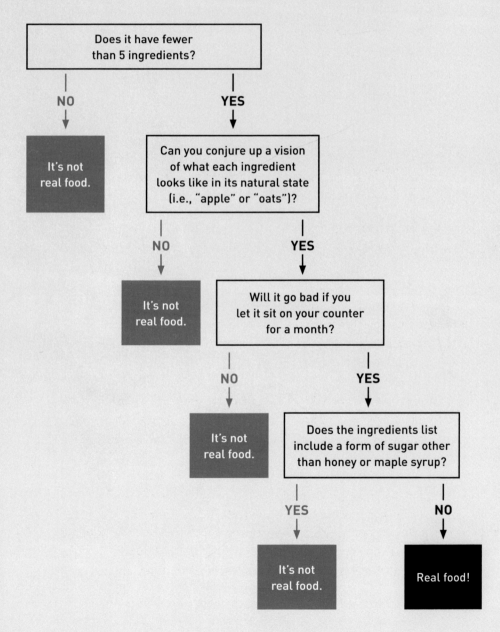

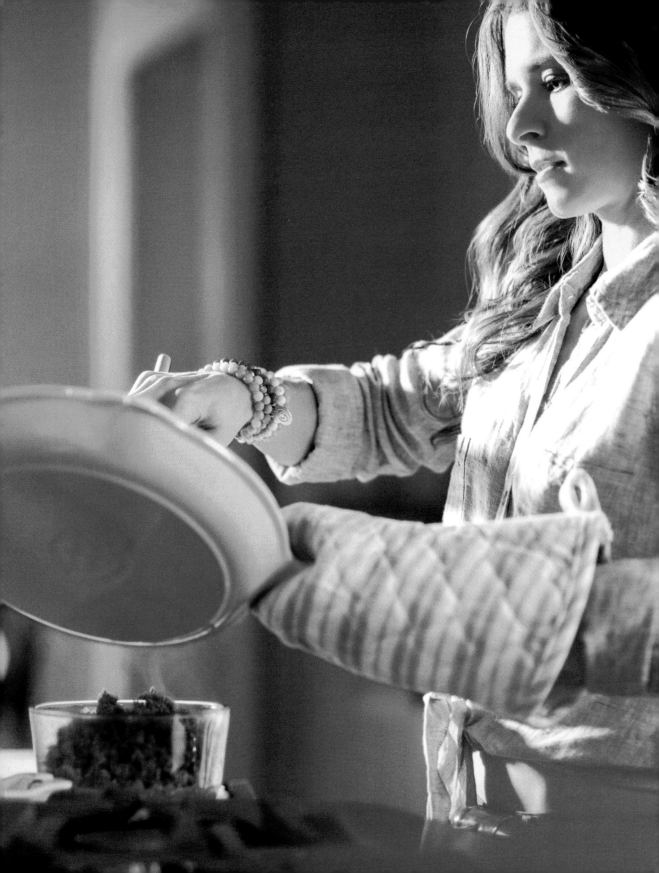

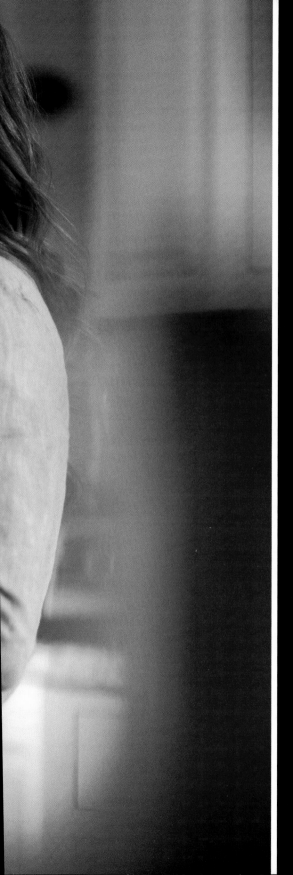

CHAPTER 13

BECOME A CHEF (YES, YOU!)

So, pretty grossed out by the last chapter?

You and me both. But hair and sand and plastic are what you're going to be eating until you take control of your food world, and the only way you are truly going to take control is to learn how to cook.

If I could give you one and only one weight-loss tip, it would be this: learn to cook at home. You can lay the foundation for the body you want in the gym, but no amount of intensity is going to overcome a poor diet.

Becoming a chef—and, yes, you can do this—will pay off in many, many ways. You will eat at home more, which is great for the waistline *and* the bottom line. You will also become so, so, so much smarter when you go out to eat. You will know why something "tastes so much better when I go out." In most cases, it's because restaurants heap tons of salt, fat, and sugar onto their food, and then ply you with enormous portions. When a ten-ounce piece of salmon (instead of the six-ounce portion you'd have at home) is on your plate, and it has that great crunchy edge (pan-sautéed in butter or oil) and tastes so flavorful (lots of salt), you will know exactly why. You will learn to tell how an item is prepared just by taste, and you'll know what all that salt and fat does to your food. You'll realize that in the end, restaurant food all tastes the same, because most restaurants use the exact same tricks: fat, salt, and sugar.

> "If you don't take care of your body, where are you going to live?"
>
> —UNKNOWN

In fact, a study at Johns Hopkins found that people who cook at home not only consume less sugar and less fat when they cook, but they also consume less when they eat out! That makes total sense to me: once you understand what food is supposed to taste like, you're less likely to be fooled by restaurant shenanigans.

How Restaurants Trick Us

A piece of salmon. A salad topped with chicken. A grilled steak.

In a normal world, these would be tremendously healthy options, packed with protein and low in salt and calories, without any scary preservatives or creepy ingredients.

But in the restaurant world, healthy dishes like this get twisted into big fistfuls of salt and fat, aimed right at your belly.

Here's the difference between cooking at home versus eating out at one of these popular restaurants:

GRILLED SALMON

	CALORIES	FAT	SATURATED FAT	SODIUM
HOMEMADE (6 OUNCES)	367	22 g	4 g	109 mg
CHILI'S ANCHO SALMON	590	27 g	5 g	1,910 mg
TGI FRIDAY'S GRILLED SALMON	970	51 g	12 g	1,830 mg
CHEESECAKE FACTORY MISO SALMON	1,670	n/a*	39 g	2,420 mg

GRILLED CHICKEN BREAST WITH GREEN SALAD

	CALORIES	FAT	SATURATED FAT	SODIUM
HOMEMADE (2 CUPS)	465	9 g	2 g	100 mg
CHILI'S BONELESS BUFFALO CHICKEN SALAD	1,020	72 g	15 g	3,480 mg
TGI FRIDAY'S PECAN-CRUSTED CHICKEN SALAD	1,080	71 g	16 g	1,650 mg
CHEESECAKE FACTORY CAESAR SALAD WITH CHICKEN	1,510	n/a*	16 g	1,450 mg

GRILLED STEAK

	CALORIES	FAT	SATURATED FAT	SODIUM
HOME-COOKED SIRLOIN (7 OUNCES)	404	18 g	6 g	268 mg
CHILI'S 10-OUNCE CLASSIC SIRLOIN	820	43 g	14 g	2,230 mg
TGI FRIDAY'S NEW YORK STRIP (WITH JACK DANIEL'S GLAZE)	1,020	49 g	21.5 g	2,680 mg
CHEESECAKE FACTORY HIBACHI STEAK	1,530	n/a*	42 g	3,720 mg

* Total fat not available

To put this in perspective, if you cooked these three meals at home instead of going out to eat, you'd save yourself, on average, 2,381 calories and 6,724 mg sodium over the course of just three nights.

If you look closely, these numbers will tell you the same thing your taste buds tell you: All that sodium and saturated fat is coming from butter and salt. It's the go-to trick for restaurants that want to disguise mediocre food and make it appeal to our taste buds.

And it's partly why restaurant food all tastes the same. They use salmon, or steak, or chicken as a delivery system for fat and salt.

Open Your Taste Buds

When you cook at home, on the other hand, *you* get to choose how things taste. *You* get to experiment with flavors and techniques, and create custom meals that satisfy your desires.

And this is my point: Eating healthy is *not* boring—it is quite the opposite. The range of colors, flavors, textures, and spices you will use will please not only your eyes, but your taste buds, too. Here are my top sources of inspiration:

Use cookbooks. Recipe sites and apps are great if you know exactly what you want to make—it's easy to Google "how to grill a chicken breast" or to find an inspiring chicken recipe on Pinterest. But nothing beats perusing a cookbook—especially one with great photos and fun side notes—to spark new thoughts, or to get you to try a food or a style of preparation you've never heard of before. It is the only way you are going to learn new preparations, cook foods you never have, and season with spices that are new to you.

> "The only real stumbling block is fear of failure. In cooking you've got to have a what-the-hell attitude."
>
> —JULIA CHILD

This is how I learned. It takes some time and preparation, but the next time you make that recipe you will be able to put your own twist on it and do it a lot faster! (I've listed some of my personal sauce-splattered favorites at the back of this book.)

Watch cooking shows. Lord knows I have watched a million hours of these. I remember back when I came home from England when I was twenty years old, I was eating a lot of chicken and veggies, and watching a lot of cooking shows. I have watched them since. My love for the show *Chopped* landed me a guest spot on the show, and I actually won the competition! (Proof that all those hours of watching paid off!) Cooking shows explain exactly how the food is made, and that's a very helpful tool. Sometimes you just don't know what the heck to do with spaghetti squash or those boring Brussels sprouts. I've learned, and I will show you!

Take cooking classes. One more fun way to learn how to cook is to take actual cooking classes. This can be a great thing to do with your girlfriends or another couple, topped off with some wine and of course a meal at the end! I planned a whole trip to Napa around a two-day cooking course at the Culinary Institute of America in St. Helena. I learned how salts affect food and the basics of wine pairing. I learned how to cook with peppers and olive oils, and how to make fresh pizza on the grill. It's probably the least likely way you will learn, but it's a good time if you make a vacation out of it!

Make Your Kitchen a Sacred Space

If you have the space, time, and money, go ahead and deck out your kitchen any way you want. A big ceiling rack filled with shiny copper pans, a little herb garden in the window, a collection of gadgets so high-tech that your countertop looks like it's ready for the Food Network. If it makes you feel at home, terrific!

Last year I splurged on my longtime kitchen dream: a La Cornue stove. Just looking at it makes me want to cook. But for much of my life I've made do with whatever was already installed in the house or apartment I was staying in. I feel confident that if I walk into anyone's home and can find a frying pan and a knife, I can make a great dinner.

My point is, you don't need to spend a ton of dough, or have a massive array of tools, to cook like a pro. Here are the essentials I recommend:

• **A high-speed blender.** If your blender can't turn ice into snow fast, it can't handle all the tasks you're going to want it to tackle. Look for one that has a wide mouth, for easy blending and cleaning, and a pulse feature. This may be the most expensive item you buy for your kitchen—a good one can cost as much as a smartphone— but a great blender can double as a food processor and wind up saving you money in the end.

- **A slow cooker.** If you have a busy life, a slow cooker will be your best friend. Sear your favorite meat in a frying pan, toss it into the slow cooker with some spices and vegetables, then go to work. When you get home, magic will be waiting.

- **A great chef's knife.** A solid, sharp chef's knife will make your kitchen prep so much easier.

- **Cast-iron skillet.** Cast iron is best because it actually imparts a tiny bit of iron into your food as you cook, which is particularly good for women, as we tend to be low on this mineral. If you can't find cast iron, look for a good heavy pan that's not coated with nonstick chemicals. (Because guess what they impart into your food?)

- **A big pot to boil in.** Big enough to cook enough chili or soup for your whole family.

- **A spatula.** I designed one for Williams-Sonoma each of the last two years to help raise money for No Kid Hungry, so if you need one, you can feed yourself and someone in need with one purchase!

- **Tongs.** Use them for everything from turning meat to serving salad. Just make sure that if they touch any uncooked meat, you clean them before using them on another part of your meal.

Reliable Partners

A short list of real foods that will last a long time.

- Apples
- Bacon/prosciutto
- Carrots, parsnips, turnips
- Citrus fruits
- Eggs
- Garlic
- Nuts, seeds, and nut butters
- Onions
- Potatoes
- Squashes

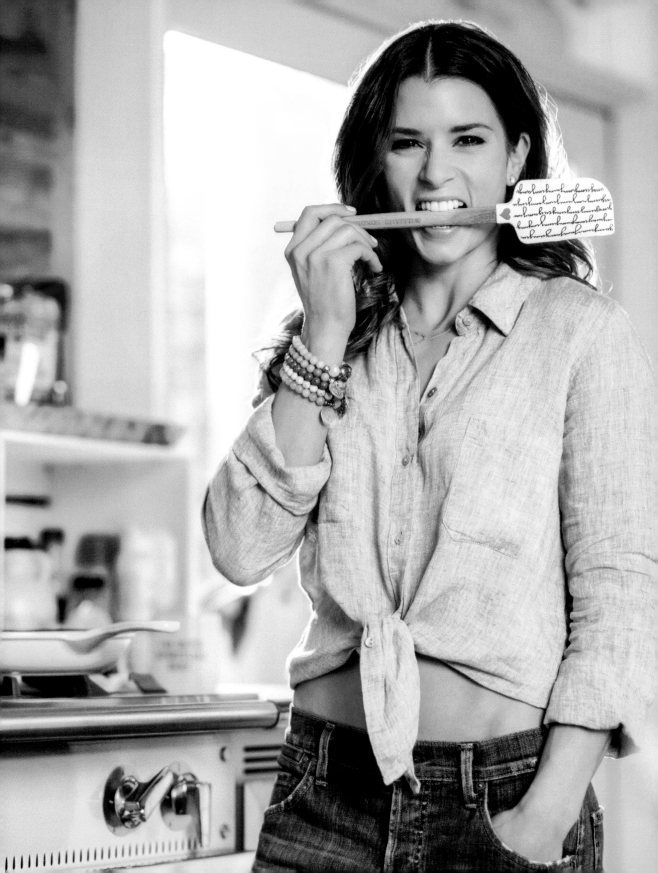

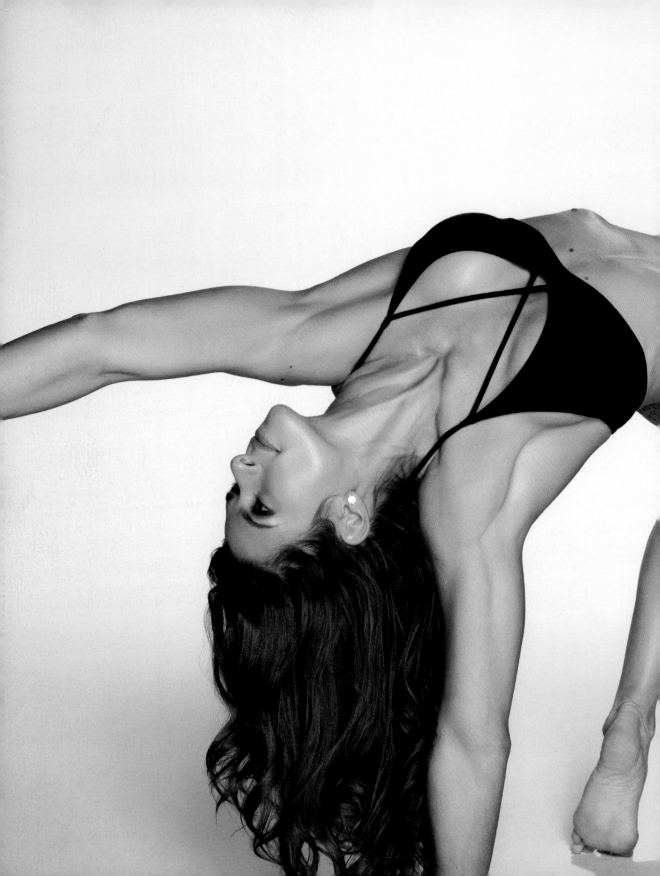

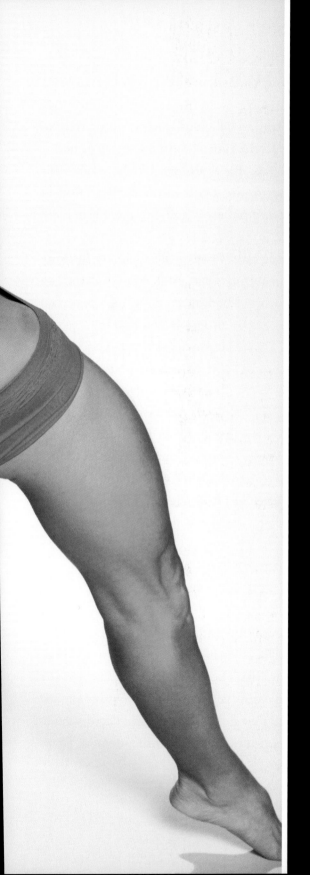

CHAPTER 14

BE
DARING
WITH
SPICES
AND FATS

A cook without an arsenal of spices and perfectly paired fats is like an artist without paint or brushes!

If you want to take food from bland to delicious, you are going to have to step outside the familiar. I'm still learning all the time about new spices or herbs, and how to pair them with the appropriate fats. It's a process, but hopefully this chapter will ignite some curiosity in you and inspire a trip to the spice section of your grocery. Just a small investment in time and money is going to pay off in a big way.

I remember when I took my first real cooking class. It was at the Culinary Institute of America (CIA) in St. Helena, California, many years ago. And, wow, I learned so much about how simple things in the kitchen could become so powerful when used properly. For example, salt: I learned how much it opened up the flavors of foods. I learned how many different flavors olive oil can have, and how to use spice taken from peppers. (Of course, the most fun was tasting wine with simple foods like a strawberry, salt, lemon, or avocado to experience just how effective pairings are, but that's for another chapter of another book!) For now, let's look a little deeper at what we are working with.

> "Cooking is like love. It should be entered into with abandon or not at all."
>
> —HARRIET VAN HORNE

Herbal Therapy

Most spices don't taste great on their own. I love biting into some wild peppermint or wintergreen if I see it growing by my house, but have you ever chewed on a sprig of rosemary or gnawed a cinnamon stick? Not so great. That's because most spices are actually a plant's version of chemical weapons: Their flavors are generated by chemicals designed to protect the plant from insects and fungi, and they don't have complex flavor profiles the way fruits do; the primary compound in mint is menthol; in thyme, thymol. So we use them in small doses, and we get big results.

Curry, turmeric, smoked paprika, pink Himalayan salt, cumin, ghee, coconut oil . . . ever heard of these, or used them? Flavors like these are going to change your life.

That's not just in the kitchen, by the way. Spices improve your health by making real food taste better, but they also have specific health benefits of their own. In one study, people were shown how to use spices in place of salt. After, the subjects were able to cut their sodium use by an average of almost 1,000 milligrams a day. That's the equivalent of five servings of Pringles! More than that, it's the difference between what most Americans consume (about 3,300 mg) and what doctors recommend (about 2,400 mg). And I don't have to tell you that too much sodium plays havoc with your blood pressure.

Flavors are chemicals, but maybe we ought to think of them as medicines. Here are some of the particular benefits you're getting from spices while your tongue is doing a happy dance:

- **Turmeric:** Helps to reduce inflammation and turns off the actions of the genes responsible for obesity.

- **Horseradish:** Turns off the action of genes responsible for growing new fat cells.

- **Black pepper:** Reduces depression, inflammation, and arthritis; improves the skin's ability to tan without burning.

- **Cinnamon:** Improves insulin response and protects against diabetes.

- **Dill, fennel, mint:** Combat digestive issues.

- **Oregano:** Helps to reduce fever, congestion, and achiness.

- **Cayenne:** May improve circulation and metabolism.

- **Mustard seeds, garlic, rosemary:** Contain antioxidants that slow aging and may help to combat cancer.

Now, overhauling your pantry with new and fresh spices and cooking fats is not going to be the cheapest thing, but it will make the simplest food amazing. The first thing you should do, however, is pull out all those little bottles you've accumulated and toss anything you don't remember buying because it was too long ago. Here are the general shelf lives of spices and herbs:

- Whole spices and dried herbs, leaves, and flowers: 1 to 2 years
- Seeds (fennel, sesame): 2 to 3 years
- Whole roots and rhizomes (such as ginger): 3 years
- Ground spices and herb leaves: 1 year
- Ground roots and rhizomes (such as ground ginger): 2 years

Some of the flavors that I've fallen in love with: Sweet potato toast with Madagascar vanilla ghee. Ground turkey with curry. Pulled pork with smoked paprika. Butternut squash roasted in coconut oil. They're just suggestions, of course: I will help you understand what goes with what generally, but your kitchen is your own playground, so go ahead and mess around!

> "Creativity is allowing yourself to make mistakes. Art is knowing which ones to keep."
>
> —SCOTT ADAMS

Let's talk about salt for a moment. I used to be very light-handed until I went to the CIA and realized how powerful it can be—if you use the right kind. Today I almost never use traditional table salt; I've moved on to kosher salt and sea salt. If you want to be flashy you can get pink Himalayan, fleur de sel, or flaky sea salt . . . just not table salt. Table salt is bland and plain because it's processed; its natural minerals have been stripped away so what's left is pure sodium chloride. It can also come in iodized form, in which iodine is added to the salt. Either way, it's not natural, and definitely missing the distinctive flavors of the minerals that occur naturally in higher-quality salts.

Eat While You Cook!

You'll find that when a new recipe doesn't taste quite right, you can save it with some combination of salt, spice, acid, sweetener, or rich fats. Promise, I do it all the time.

That's why you have to taste your food as you go. *Have to!* I probably taste and balance flavors at least three or four times. It's an art, which means there is no wrong, just what you like!

If a dish tastes bland, use this cheat sheet to help get it up on its feet.

THE FOOD	THE SPICES AND FATS
PORK	Salt, pepper, rosemary, thyme, mustard, paprika, onion powder, garlic powder, cinnamon, ghee, avocado oil, olive oil, sage
FISH	Salt, pepper, paprika, coriander, onion powder, avocado oil, ghee, ginger, dill, cilantro
RED MEATS	Salt, pepper, oregano, thyme, rosemary, coconut sugar, onion powder, garlic powder, olive oil
VEGETABLES	Salt, pepper, paprika, curry, turmeric, oregano, chives, garlic powder, onion powder, lemon, rosemary, thyme, cayenne, ghee, avocado oil, olive oil
SWEETS AND DESSERTS	Salt, cinnamon, nutmeg, cardamom, vanilla, balsamic, maple syrup, honey, cloves, ginger

Put Your Herb Garden to Work

Most of the herbs and spices you'll use throughout the year are dried, but don't forget about the real power of fresh herbs like thyme, rosemary, basil, parsley, mint, and cilantro. There are so many variations that I am learning about right now since I planted a big garden right outside my kitchen door. If you can grow herbs in your backyard, on your porch, or on a windowsill, they'll help keep your kitchen tasting, and smelling, great all year. Here's what to do with them:

- **Basil**: Meat, vegetables, fruit
- **Cilantro**: Fish, vegetables
- **Mint**: Vegetables, fruit
- **Parsley**: Fish, vegetables, fruit
- **Rosemary**: Meat, poultry, pork, fruit, vegetables
- **Thyme**: Meat, poultry, pork, vegetables

How to Live More Richly

I hope that by the time you've arrived at this chapter, you're already convinced that the old saying "You are what you eat" doesn't apply to fat. The fat we eat helps support our endocrine system, keeps us full, and plays a huge role in a number of body functions, from muscle building to fat burning.

And fortunately, the healthiest fats are also the tastiest. These oils are all rich in heart-healthy omega-3 fatty acids, monounsaturated fats, and lauric acid (all good for you), and contain lower levels of omega-6 fatty acids (which we eat too much of). The right balance of fats will help control inflammation, making weight loss easier, while taking your taste buds on the ride of their lives!

Cross these off your shopping list: corn oil, sunflower oil, soybean oil, "vegetable" oil (it's usually made from soybeans), palm oil, and safflower oil. They're all cheap oils that are primarily made up of inflammation-boosting omega-6 fatty acids.

CANOLA OIL

Why It's Healthy: Ever eaten a canola? You sorta have, if you've eaten broccoli; canola oil comes from the seeds of a plant in the broccoli family, and it's a great source of omega-3 fats. A study review in *Experimental Biology and Medicine* found that people who achieve a balance of omega-3s similar to that found in canola oil are better able to ward off cancer, arthritis, and asthma. It's also rich in alpha-linolenic acid (ALA), an essential omega-3 fatty acid that may help control weight, according to a study in the *Journal of Functional Foods*.

How to Use It: For everyday cooking, canola oil is your best choice. It's flavor-neutral (so you won't taste it as strongly as olive or coconut oil), and it can withstand very high levels of heat. Use canola oil in place of vegetable oil and you'll make an enormous impact on your health.

COCONUT OIL

Why It's Healthy: It's a great source of lauric acid, a medium-chain saturated fat that your body can convert into energy more easily than other types of fat.

How to Use It: Anytime you'd normally reach for butter—for example, to fry some eggs—try reaching for coconut oil instead. It tastes great drizzled over sweet potato hash browns, and it's terrific for frying chicken breasts.

AVOCADO OIL

Why It's Healthy: A top source of heart-healthy monounsaturated fats that help raise your "good" cholesterol and keep you feeling full. Avocado is rich in vitamins B and E and potassium, and it's one of the top go-to fats for people following a Paleo diet.

How to Use It: Like a salad oil, or drizzled over fish. It also pairs nicely with tomatoes, watermelon, grapefruit, and oranges.

GHEE

Why It's Healthy: Ghee is clarified butter, and easy to make at home. Just put some sticks of butter in a small saucepan, melt them and bring to a gentle boil, then cook over low heat until the water in the butter has evaporated and the milk solids have sunk to the bottom of the pot and browned. Skim off any foam remaining on the surface and reserve the clear yellow liquid, which you can then store in a sealed jar. Ghee is lower in lactose than whole butter, and rich in butyrate, a fatty acid that's linked to decreased inflammation.

How to Use It: Any way that you'd use butter; you'll get all the flavor but little if any of the lactose.

MACADAMIA NUT OIL

Why It's Healthy: It's hard to find, but macadamia nut oil is 84 percent monounsaturated and super-rich in omega-3 fatty acids. It's also a source of phytosterols, compounds associated with decreased cancer risk.

How to Use It: Try using it in baking, stir-frying, and oven cooking. Toss slices of sweet potatoes with the nut oil and bake in a preheated oven at 350°F for 20 minutes or until crispy.

OLIVE OIL

Why It's Healthy: Extra-virgin olive oil may increase your levels of serotonin, a hormone associated with happiness. It's also a source of antiaging compounds called polyphenols, which help improve bone strength and brain function.

How to Use It: Use the expensive extra-virgin stuff for dressing salads, vegetables, and cooked foods. When you're using olive oil to cook with (and it's really versatile), go ahead and use the less-expensive regular or light versions.

WALNUT OIL

Why It's Healthy: Walnut oil can actually help your body respond better to stress and keep its blood pressure steady, according to a study at Penn State. Walnut oil is also rich in certain types of polyunsaturated fatty acids that have been shown to increase calorie burn and boost metabolism. And walnuts are richer in omega-3 fatty acids than any other nut.

How to Use It: Use it in place of extra-virgin olive oil for an extra nutty kick. You can make a quick salad dressing by mixing it with balsamic vinegar and a pinch of sea salt.

FLAXSEED OIL

Why It's Healthy: Flaxseed is packed with ALA, an omega-3 fatty acid that helps keep your weight stable, reduces inflammation, and keeps your blood vessels healthy.

How to Use It: You can't really cook with flaxseed oil, although you can add it to baking recipes that call for vegetable oil. Try using it instead of olive oil or mayo when whipping up sauces, pesto, or a tuna salad.

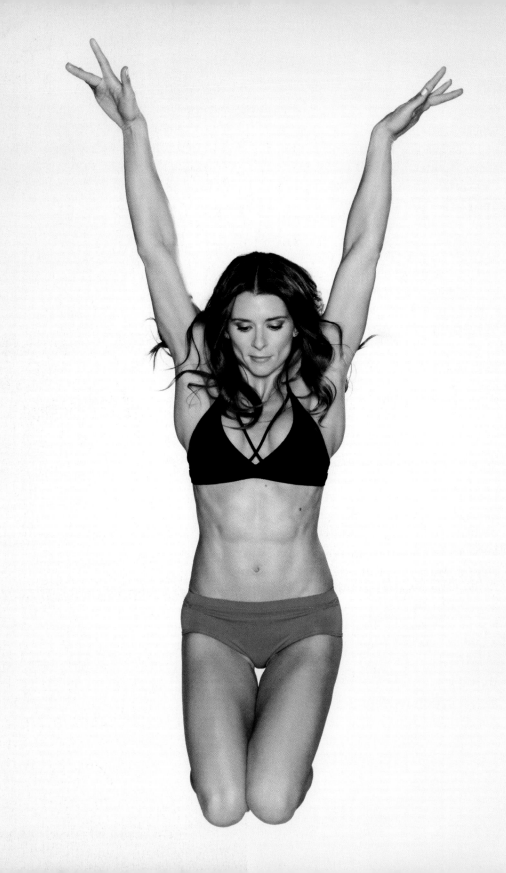

CHAPTER 15

BURN YOUR FOOD

Why are junk foods so popular, so hard to resist, even when we know how bad they are for us? In a lot of cases, it comes down to one word: *Crunch.*

After all, potato chips and nachos and crackers and Cheez Doodles and all those other salty snacks you can't eat just one of all have something in common, and that's crispiness. Compare that to boiled broccoli or steamed squash or any other mushy vegetable your mom used to force you to eat, and it's no wonder the fried foods win out. So instead of trying to convince you that steamed Brussels sprouts are delicious, I'm going to show you how to make healthy foods tastier, sexier . . . and yes, crunchier.

I am as serious about food presentation as I am about the actual preparation. There is such a big difference between mushy, warmed-up Brussels sprouts and sprouts that are perfectly crisped and charred. There is a difference between an overcooked steak and one that melts in your mouth and still has those beautiful #hashmarks.

This chapter will teach you to turn ordinary meats and vegetables into something that tastes like it came straight from Bobby Flay's kitchen.

Why We Crave the Crunch

When man first tamed fire, it meant he could now cook and eat the meat from the animals he hunted. (Before we learned to cook our food, all we could eat were the gross soft bits like innards, eyes, and brains!) And he could eat a wider variety of vegetation as well, since fire could break up the thick, fibrous parts of otherwise inedible foods like squash. Suddenly, an enormous amount of nutrition became available to us. So it's no wonder we're driven to seek out crunchy foods; when we bite into something crisp, our ancient brains are triggered to anticipate a nutritious feast (instead of just "Ugh, liver again!").

Scientists claim that we like crunchy foods because they enhance the sensory experience of eating. A piece of meat blackened on the grill simply smells richer than one from the oven. And crispy foods not only stimulate our senses of taste and smell; they also feel more interesting in our mouths.

And don't forget that beyond taste, smell, and feel, there's another sense that's stimulated by food: sound. Sizzle, pop, crunch. It's just more interesting than the slurp of soup, no? Scientists have recently discovered proteins that influence both our sense of taste and our hearing, and speculate that certain foods excite our brains by stimulating both senses simultaneously.

From Roasting to Boasting

Scientists call it the Maillard effect: It's what happens when the proteins and carbohydrates in our food react to intense heat to turn brown on the outside and release their full flavor and aroma. So consider these tips the keys to maximum Maillard:

RULE #1: Get your food warm before you get it hot.
Few things make me as sad as watching someone pull a gorgeous steak out of the fridge and flop it onto a grill.

Food wasn't meant to be cooked cold. In the refrigerator, the fibers of the food tighten up. When you put cold food onto a hot grill, the fibers expand as the food is cooking, meaning that parts of the food cook more than other parts. You also have to wait for the grill, oven, or pan to heat the whole piece of meat through, so in turn you overcook the outside, making it tough and dry.

This is especially important with protein. People tell me my steak is one of the top five steaks they have ever had. It's not because I use some special seasoning or unhealthy add-in, it is because I leave my steaks on the counter for at least an hour before I cook them. Your protein is the most important thing to warm up because it is normally very dense and thick compared to a vegetable.

RULE #2: Blot.
Water is the enemy of crispiness. Whether you're pan-frying chicken, grilling steak, or sautéing vegetables, wetness on the surface of the food will keep the exterior from browning up. If you are roasting or sautéing something, the water needs to cook off before your food can caramelize, brown, and develop intense flavors. Some foods, such as onions or mushrooms, need to be given time to dry after they're cut; others, such as a whole chicken, can be blotted; and shredded foods can be squeezed out.

RULE #3: Give it some space.

You are not making a casserole here, you are trying to capture that brown, caramel exterior. To do that, you want heat to circulate around your food evenly. If your food is all on top of itself, it will not brown the way you want it to.

I use multiple pans or trays to make sure all the food has contact with the cooking surface. Food cooks faster when it is touching the highest point of heat. I know, sometimes it's tempting to squeeze everything into one pan or oven rack to save cleanup on the back end. But there's a golden rule of doing dishes: the more delicious the meal, the less painful the cleanup. (Well, at least I wish that were the case!)

RULE #4: Be patient.

By "patient," I don't mean low and slow, either. I mean turn that damn timer off and use your eyes and cooking utensils to see when things are ready. If you are roasting or grilling something, check to see if you are getting char marks; meat won't even come off the pan or grill until it has browned. If your meat sticks and gets messed, that's okay.

Now, I know a lot of times people worry about leaving their protein undercooked, so here are some food-safety tips to make sure you're in the clear:

Steak: Don't cut into it! You'll lose the essential juiciness. Instead, using your tongs, poke the meat right in the middle, on the top. If it is very squishy, it is not done. If it is very firm, it's overcooked. You want it to be a little soft in the middle for medium-well and a little soft from edge to edge for medium-rare.

Pork and Chicken: They need to be cooked through, but they should not be totally firm, or the cuts will be very dry and overdone. You want something that squishes just a little when you poke it with your utensil.

Fish: I like to wrap fish in aluminum foil and make an enclosed package with it to keep the moisture in and eliminate the challenge of having to flip it. When you see white start to push out of the fish, it is almost overdone. That is the only visual aid I know. A fish is done perfectly when it's no longer opaque in the middle.

People are always blown away when I don't set a timer for anything I am cooking. I am sure you too have been there when you are cooking a recipe according to what's stated in the directions, but when that time is up, you're convinced that it's not done. Well, you're right. Trust your instincts!

There are too many variables that go into cooking for you not to be patient and wait for the food to be what you want it to be. That recipe might not be accurate: Who knows what temperature the food was when it went into the pan or oven or on the grill? Who knows how your cooking appliance puts off heat, or what kind of pan you are using, or if you are the type who keeps opening the oven to "check on dinner"? These are all variables that never make it into the cookbooks. So, in the recipe section of this book, I have given you estimated cooking times, but they are just suggestions. Only you can determine when something is "done."

HOW TO PREPARE ANY VEGETABLE

THE VEGGIE	THE TIME	THE METHOD	
ZUCCHINI OR SUMMER SQUASH	6 to 8 minutes each side	Grill	Don't try to cut your squash into little circles or they'll all wind up as little charcoal hockey pucks at the bottom of the grate. Cut them lengthwise, about ¼ inch thick.
ONIONS	12 to 15 minutes each side	Grill or sauté	Another vegetable that's famous for turning into burnt offerings at the bottom of the grill. Instead, peel the onion, slice it into ¼-inch-thick pieces, and skewer them together with toothpicks. Grill for 3 to 5 minutes and then flip them over. If you want the onion to really caramelize, cook it at a lower temperature for at least 30 minutes.
EGGPLANT	6 to 8 minutes each side	Grill	Eggplant is a very dry vegetable, so make sure you rub it with olive oil or avocado oil first.
CARROTS	40 to 60 minutes	Roast	If the carrots are thick, cut them in half lengthwise. Try spicing them up with some Middle Eastern spices like cumin or coriander, as well as salt and pepper. I have always found carrots to take a long time to caramelize and brown. I roast them for up to 1 hour.
BROCCOLI OR CAULIFLOWER	10 to 15 minutes	Roast	Roasting these vegetables offers so much potential for extra crunch because of all the edges on them!
ASPARAGUS	15 to 20 minutes	Grill	Make sure you line up the asparagus perpendicular to the grill grates so they don't slip through. Did I really need to say that?!
BELL PEPPERS	8 to 10 minutes	Grill	Cut the pepper so there is as much surface as possible touching the grill. Remove the seeds and stems. I usually end up with about four chunks per pepper.

General Guideline Temperatures for Each Preparation Technique:
Grill: 350–400°F • Oven: 375–425°F • Pan: Low to medium

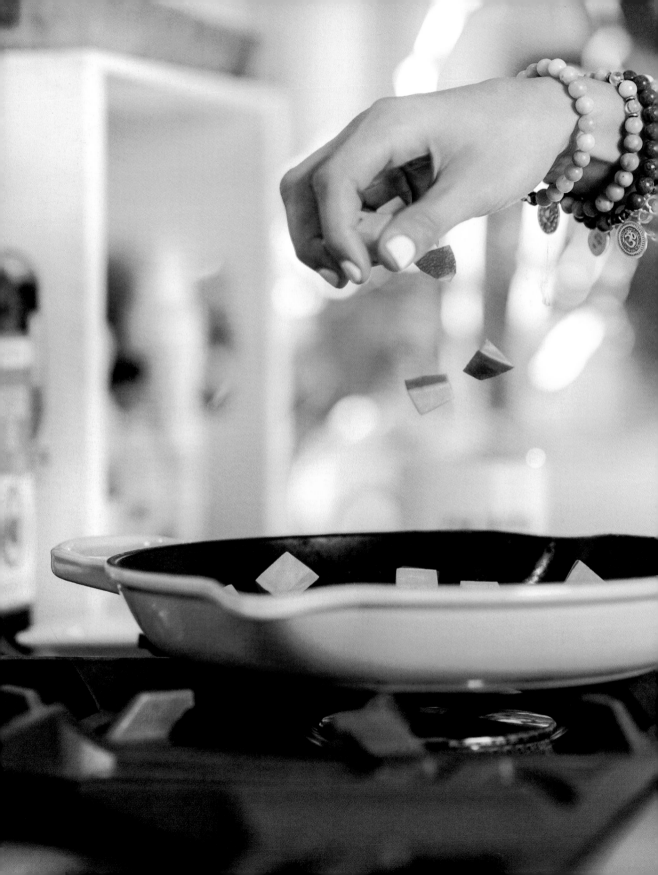

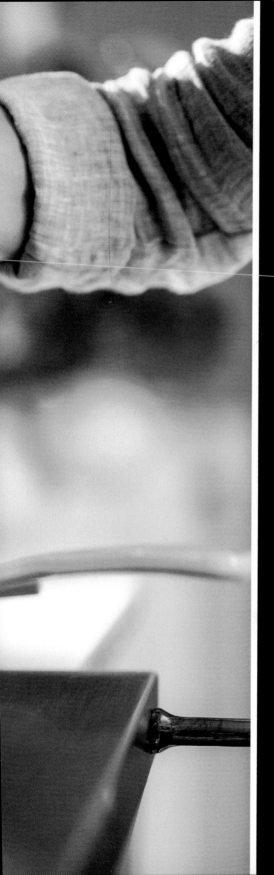

CHAPTER 16

THE COMPLETE *PRETTY INTENSE* FOODS PLAN

To help your body start burning fat and give you the energy you need, the *Pretty Intense* nutrition plan focuses on a series of super-healthy food groups, each of which spark metabolism in its own particular way, while giving your overall health a boost:

EAT MORE: **Meat (grass-fed beef, poultry, fish, and game); in your main meals**
Why? To burn fat and build lean muscle.

Lean meat helps burn fat in a number of ways. First, it takes the body more energy to burn off a gram of protein than a gram of carbohydrate. This is known as the "thermogenic effect of digestion." Eating 100 calories' worth of protein simply isn't the same as eating 100 calories' worth of carbs: your body burns off 20 to 30 percent of protein calories you eat just by digesting it; it only uses 5 to 10 percent of the carb calories you eat for digestion. That's just one reason why studies have shown that when subjects are put on high-protein diets versus high-carbohydrate diets, the high-protein groups lose more weight—even if the number of calories they eat is exactly the same. And high-protein diets are also linked repeatedly to lower triglyceride levels, blood pressure, and waist circumference.

> "The only time to eat diet food is while you're waiting for the steak to cook."
>
> —JULIA CHILD

EAT MORE: **Vegetables (any); as often as you want**
Why? Because you'll fill your body with the nutrients it needs for almost zero calories.

By vegetables, I mean brightly colored green, red, yellow, and purple vegetables: carrots, tomatoes, celery, lettuce, squash, and leafy greens. This is what you need to pack vitamins, minerals, and fiber into your body with a minimum of calories. What's not included in this list are fries and chips, and starchy beans, peas, and lentils.

I make sure I eat vegetables at every meal. I'll toss some spinach in with my eggs or shred up a sweet potato for a breakfast hash; whip up a salad with some protein for lunch; and make sure vegetables are the visual bulk of what fills me up at dinnertime. Consider this: Those who eat eight or more servings of fruits and vegetables a day are 30 percent less likely to suffer a heart attack or stroke.

EAT MORE: Fruits (lean toward lower glycemic options—berries, melons, citrus, apples)

Why? For maximum energy and a huge dose of nutrition.

What if you could strip off more than a dozen pounds of fat simply by buying a bunch of fruit and putting it in a bowl on your kitchen table?

In a study at Cornell University, researchers photographed more than two hundred kitchens, and then weighed the people who owned them. They discovered that what sits out in your kitchen can have a huge influence on your weight. People who had breakfast cereal sitting out on their counters weighed about twenty pounds more than average; those with soda sitting out in the kitchen weighed between twenty-four and twenty-six pounds more. But those who had a bowl of fruit sitting out weighed, on average, thirteen pounds less than the average person.

The reason is that we eat what we see, and when you're constantly confronted with fruit, you're bound to eat more of it, and that's a terrific way to reshape your body for the better. Dark fruits (and vegetables) have higher levels of nutrients called flavonoids, which give plants their color. In a study of about 250,000 people, those with the highest intake of flavonoid-rich foods gained the least amount of weight over a period of twenty-four years.

EAT MORE: Nuts, seeds, and healthy fats; throughout the day

Why? Because they ward off hunger.

Just about every nutrient you need for health—vitamins, minerals, protein, fiber, and healthy fats—are found in nuts and seeds. They're like little weight-loss pills. A review of studies in the *American Journal of Clinical Nutrition* found that consuming nuts could help ward off weight gain, protect against heart disease, and lower diabetes risk. (While all nuts and seeds are healthy, walnuts in particular are associated with a reduced likelihood of diabetes.) But look for raw nuts; the "roasted and salted" versions are often roasted in unhealthy oils, and the additional sodium isn't anything you need.

EAT MORE: Eggs

Why? For great protein and satisfying fat to get your metabolism revving.

I eat eggs almost every morning. One egg has about 70 calories but provides 6 grams of protein and zero carbs, and half of the fat in an egg is heart-healthy monounsaturated fat. Plus, eggs are the best dietary source of choline, a nutrient that's essential for keeping our metabolism running hot. Most Americans don't get enough of this B vitamin, for good reason: the best sources are raw beef liver, cauliflower, codfish oil, and brewer's yeast. Yum! One egg contains a third of the 425 mg adults should consume every day. You'd have to eat a pound of cauliflower to get as much choline as you'll get from one egg!

But what about the cholesterol? Even if cholesterol is a problem for you, eating eggs—or other nutritious foods that are high in cholesterol, like shrimp—needn't be a concern. Health experts no longer consider cholesterol from the foods we eat to be a main cause of high cholesterol in our bloodstreams, and even the US government, which does everything under the yellow caution flag, now says that cholesterol in food isn't a concern.

What is a concern is making sure you get enough protein at breakfast to jump-start your metabolism. That's why eggs are such a huge part of my morning routine. If you don't care for eggs, consider starting your morning with ground meats like beef, bison, or turkey.

Foods to Avoid

The plan specifically eliminates gluten and dairy. They are inflammatory foods and also disrupt the gut more than any other food groups. Please do your best to take them out of your diet along with processed fats and sugars, and see how great you feel!

AVOID: Refined flour-based foods (any items that contain gluten)
Why? Because you'll store less fat and experience less fatigue.

You've been told about the importance of whole grains for so long that you're probably going back and double-checking right now: "Does Danica really want me to avoid cereal, bread, and pasta?"

The answer is yes. Because when you eliminate grains, you eliminate those three-P.M. bouts of fatigue and sugar cravings so many of us struggle with.

Once I cut grains out of my daily diet, I discovered I no longer felt hungry or tired during the day. And that's what you'll experience, too: the end of "low energy" days.

You will also experience far less discomfort after eating a meal. If I eat right, I never feel "full," just satisfied.

AVOID: Animal-based dairy (including yogurt, milk, and cheese)

Why? Because you'll reduce inflammation and flatten your belly, fast.

You've heard of lactose intolerance, of course: that's the inability to digest lactose, a sugar found in milk and other dairy products. But even if you don't have a full-blown lactose intolerance, you'll find that by eliminating dairy from your diet, you'll feel leaner and cleaner all day, every day.

The bloating that dairy causes comes from a disturbance in our gut bacteria. (Yes, we all have them—about five hundred different species, some good and some bad, living in our digestive tract.) Dairy products disrupt the natural balance of bacteria in the belly, potentially leading to what's known as a "leaky gut." (That's when the lining of your digestive tract becomes inflamed, allowing toxins to leak into your body from your intestines. It's an extremely common problem.)

AVOID: Soy-based foods and soybean, corn, or vegetable oil

Why? Because you'll cut down on fat storage and inflammation.

Soybeans have a lot of good stuff in them, especially protein and fiber. But the vast majority of soy we eat doesn't come in the form of those simple beans; it comes in the form of processed, concentrated stuff like soybean oil (used in everything from salad dressings to French fries to muffins). And that's where we start to run into trouble. Processed soy is very high in two things you want to avoid: omega-6 fatty acids, which increase inflammation throughout your body, and estrogenic chemicals, which trigger your body to store fat. While an occasional serving of edamame or miso soup won't hurt, avoid anything that's made with "vegetable oil" (which usually means soybean oil), and use olive oil, avocado oil, or coconut oil for your home cooking.

AVOID: Sugar

Why? Because you'll reduce hunger and your risk of disease.

If I could get you to take away one single piece of healthy eating advice, it would be this: Cut down on sugar.

Sugar feeds the unhealthy bacteria in your body, leading to everything from belly bloating to cavities. Sugar supresses a key immune response known as phagocytosis. Cancer cells feed on sugar! Sugar drives your insulin levels crazy, leading to fat storage and rebound hunger. New research shows that sugar even interferes with the body's ability to synthesize protein—meaning it makes your muscles smaller, reducing your metabolic rate and undermining all the hard work you do in the gym.

Foods to Cut Down On

These foods can be part of your regular diet, but they're not as healthy for you as you might think. In fact, they probably do more harm than good.

CUT DOWN ON: Beans, lentils, peanuts, and other legumes
Why? Because they undermine your nutritional goals.

Brown rice and beans used to be a staple of my diet. And why not? We've been told over and over again how healthy and nutritious this pairing is, especially if we're trying to cut down on fat.

But while beans and other legumes (legumes are anything that comes in a pod, like peanuts, lentils, peas, chickpeas, or soybeans) do have some protein and fiber, they're much heavier in starch—and should be considered more like grains than the little protein-and-fiber superfoods we often think of them as. They also contain a compound called phytic acid, which binds to the nutrients in food, preventing your body from accessing them. So while it may seem you're getting plenty of protein and other nutrients from beans, the truth is less rosy than you think. For that reason, it's okay to have the occasional bean dip, but don't make beans a major part of your diet, and swap out peanut butter for healthier options like almond or cashew butter.

CUT DOWN ON: Gluten-free grains (rice, oats, quinoa)
Why? Because they're packed with empty calories.

But wait: You've been told so often about the importance of fiber!

Whether it's "whole grain," "steel cut," "unrefined," "gluten free," or whatever terms that make those grains seem so healthy and enticing, the fact is that when you eat grains, you're still getting a food that's relatively high in empty calories and low in nutrients—including fiber. A woman would have to eat 7 cups of brown rice (about 1,500 calories worth) or 13 slices of whole-grain bread (more than 1,000 calories) or 14 ears of corn (about 850 calories) every day to get the 25 grams of fiber recommended by the USDA.

But eat the way I do, with fruit and vegetables at every meal instead of grains, and look what happens: 2 apples, a cup of blueberries, a peach, a cup of broccoli, a serving of romaine lettuce, and a handful (about ⅓ cup) of almonds gets you to 25 grams of fiber for just 714 calories, and you're also getting a wide array of vitamins and minerals as well as some healthy fats and protein. Have vegetables at every meal, snack on fruit and nuts throughout the day, and you don't need to eat grains. You'll still be getting the fiber your body needs to stay lean: in one study of more than 1,100 people over five years, researchers found that for every 10 grams of fiber people ate, their belly fat accumulation was reduced by nearly 4 percent—even if they did nothing else to lose weight.

By stripping away these unnecessary sources of extra calories, you'll also strip away one of the biggest causes of weight gain: insulin spikes.

Insulin is the hormone that manages blood sugar. When our bodies get a big dose of carbohydrates, we quickly digest it, turning it into sugar. (And remember, we hardly burn any calories digesting carbs, so 95 percent of those calories hit our systems, and fast!) Our pancreas then responds by creating insulin, which helps shuttle the sugar out of our blood and into our cells, where we can use it for energy. But too many carbohydrates at any one time—whether from a candy bar or a bag of pretzels or a big bowl of oatmeal—means we've got more sugar on hand than our bodies can use. Since that sugar has to go somewhere, our bodies do the simplest thing: store that sugar as fat. And once our bodies store that sugar as fat, insulin drops, causing rebound hunger, fatigue—and the search for more carbs.

Sample Shopping List

Not everything on this list may be to your liking, and you certainly won't need to buy it all, but as you plan out your next ninety days, this mix-and-match list will come in handy. Try to pick a protein and two vegetables for each meal. *Any* fruit, vegetable, meat, fish, nut, or seed is okay. This is a grocery list of my favorites.

Vegetables

- ☐ Spinach
- ☐ Kale
- ☐ Cauliflower
- ☐ Broccoli
- ☐ Brussels sprouts
- ☐ Mushrooms
- ☐ Swiss chard

- ☐ Garlic
- ☐ Red bell peppers
- ☐ Onion
- ☐ Zucchini
- ☐ Yellow squash
- ☐ Cherry tomatoes
- ☐ Cucumbers

- ☐ Celery
- ☐ Carrots
- ☐ Acorn squash
- ☐ Spaghetti squash
- ☐ Butternut squash
- ☐ Purple potatoes
- ☐ Sweet potatoes

Fruits

- ☐ Blackberries
- ☐ Raspberries
- ☐ Strawberries
- ☐ Blueberries

- ☐ Pineapple
- ☐ Bananas
- ☐ Apple
- ☐ Pears

- ☐ Limes
- ☐ Avocado
- ☐ Lemons

Dried Fruits (make sure there is no sugar added!)

- ☐ Raisins
- ☐ Mulberries

- ☐ Dates
- ☐ Figs

- ☐ Goji berries

Milk Alternatives

- ☐ Unsweetened almond milk
- ☐ Unsweetened coconut milk

- ☐ Cashew milk
- ☐ Canned full-fat coconut milk

- ☐ Canned light coconut milk

Protein

- ☐ Ground beef (grass-fed)
- ☐ Ground bison/buffalo
- ☐ Rotisserie chicken
- ☐ Ground turkey
- ☐ Whole birds (for roasting or the slow cooker)
- ☐ Eggs
- ☐ Chicken breast
- ☐ Fish (wild salmon, halibut)
- ☐ Pork roast (for the slow cooker)
- ☐ Lamb
- ☐ Bacon

Nuts/Seeds

- ☐ Walnuts
- ☐ Cashews
- ☐ Almonds (sliced, slivered, whole)
- ☐ Pecans
- ☐ Pistachios
- ☐ Chia seeds
- ☐ Sunflower seeds
- ☐ Hemp seeds
- ☐ Tahini
- ☐ Almond butter
- ☐ Cashew butter

Oils/Condiments/Ingredients

- ☐ Extra-virgin olive oil
- ☐ Coconut oil
- ☐ Avocado oil
- ☐ Ghee (clarified butter; see page 183)
- ☐ Olives (green or black)
- ☐ Dried basil, thyme, rosemary
- ☐ Ground mustard
- ☐ Cayenne pepper
- ☐ Paprika
- ☐ Garlic powder
- ☐ Balsamic vinegar (aged tastes best)
- ☐ Marinara sauce (homemade or a brand with no sugar added)
- ☐ Vanilla extract
- ☐ Coconut flakes
- ☐ Dark chocolate (72% cacao or higher)
- ☐ Almond flour
- ☐ Coconut flour
- ☐ Cocoa nibs
- ☐ Honey
- ☐ Pure maple syrup

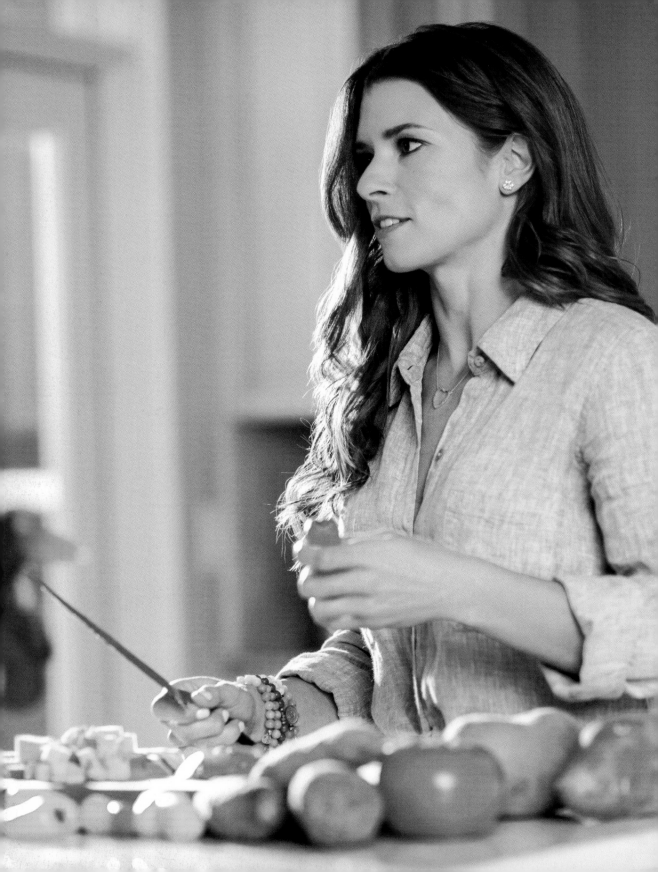

CHAPTER 17

THE *PRETTY INTENSE* RECIPES

I developed these recipes through years of tweaking, testing, and tasting before settling on the perfect combinations for myself and my family. They're the perfect recipes for us, but you might like things sweeter, or more savory, or packing a spicier punch. That's fine; as I said earlier, the kitchen is a place for you to unleash your own creativity. So consider these recipes a very solid starting point for your own edible experiments.

All that matters in the end is that you're eating *real* food, not something cooked up in a laboratory by food scientists. Almost all these recipes depend on just a handful of ingredients—food that comes from the earth or from the animals that feed from it. Just remember a few simple rules:

Eat More: Meats, fish, all vegetables including root vegetables and all squashes, fruit, nuts, seeds, coconut oil, olive oil, ghee, avocado oil, nut milks, coconut milk, sweet potatoes, and eggs

Avoid: Dairy (including milk, cheese, and yogurt), wheat flour–based foods (including whole-grain and white bread, pasta, and pastries), soy, sugar, and artificial sweeteners

Cut Down On: Legumes (peas, beans, lentils, peanuts), grains (corn, oats, rice, quinoa)

Always Eat: Breakfast, and then every three hours, especially after a workout

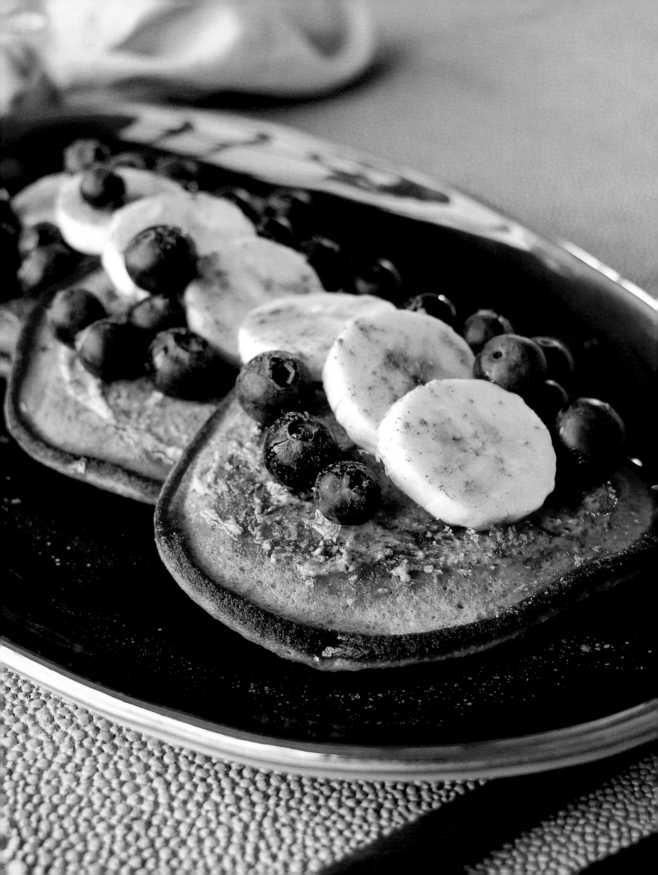

Maca Pumpkin Pancakes

MAKES 4 TO 6 PANCAKES

3 teaspoons coconut oil

2 large eggs

2 tablespoons almond flour

1 tablespoon coconut flour

¼ cup pure pumpkin

1 teaspoon maca powder

¼ teaspoon ground cinnamon

In a large sauté pan, melt 2 teaspoons of the coconut oil over medium heat, swirling the pan to coat completely. In a large bowl using a fork or whisk, mix the eggs, almond flour, coconut flour, pumpkin, maca, and cinnamon. Spoon half the batter into the pan to make 3 small pancakes. Place a fry screen over the pan to help trap the heat. Once the edges are brown and the tops of the pancakes are firm on the edges, flip the pancakes; the second side takes much less time to cook. Repeat with the remaining 1 teaspoon coconut oil and remaining batter. Top with any fruit, nut butter, honey, syrup, or butter you like. I use Madagascar vanilla ghee, almond butter, and honey, blueberries, and banana.

Simple Waffles

MAKES 8 TO 10 WAFFLES

2 tablespoons coconut oil, melted

3 large eggs

½ teaspoon pure vanilla extract

1 tablespoon honey

½ cup almond flour

½ cup coconut flour

½ teaspoon baking soda

1 cup unsweetened almond milk

Preheat your waffle maker. In a large glass bowl, stir together the coconut oil, eggs, vanilla, and honey to combine. In a separate bowl, mix the almond flour, coconut flour, and baking soda with a fork. Combine the wet and dry ingredients, then stir in the almond milk. Pour a portion of the batter into the waffle maker and cook according to the manufacturer's instructions. Transfer the waffles to a plate and keep warm in a low oven or serve immediately. Repeat with the remaining batter. If you double this recipe, adjust the almond flour to 1¼ cups and the coconut flour to ¾ cup.

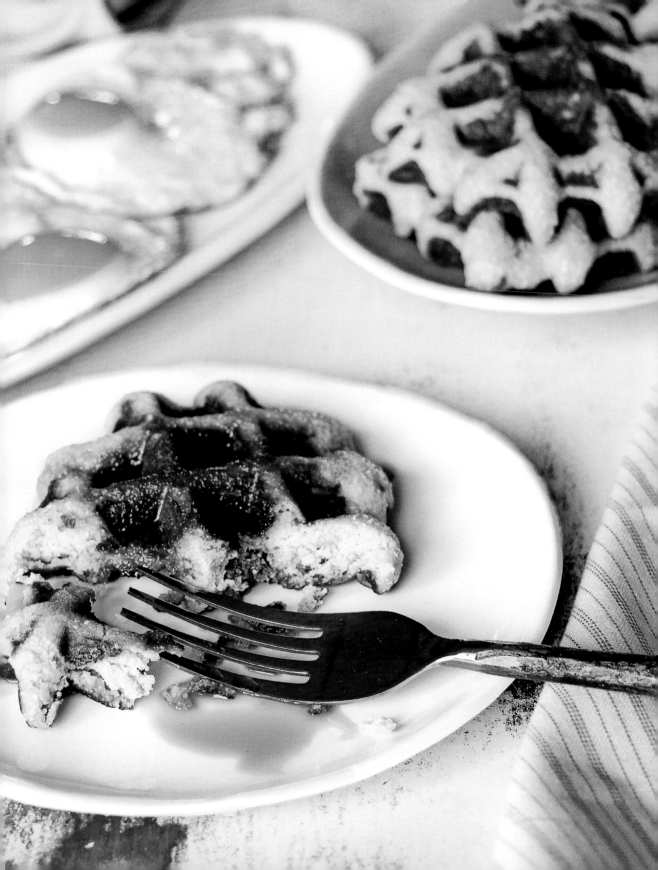

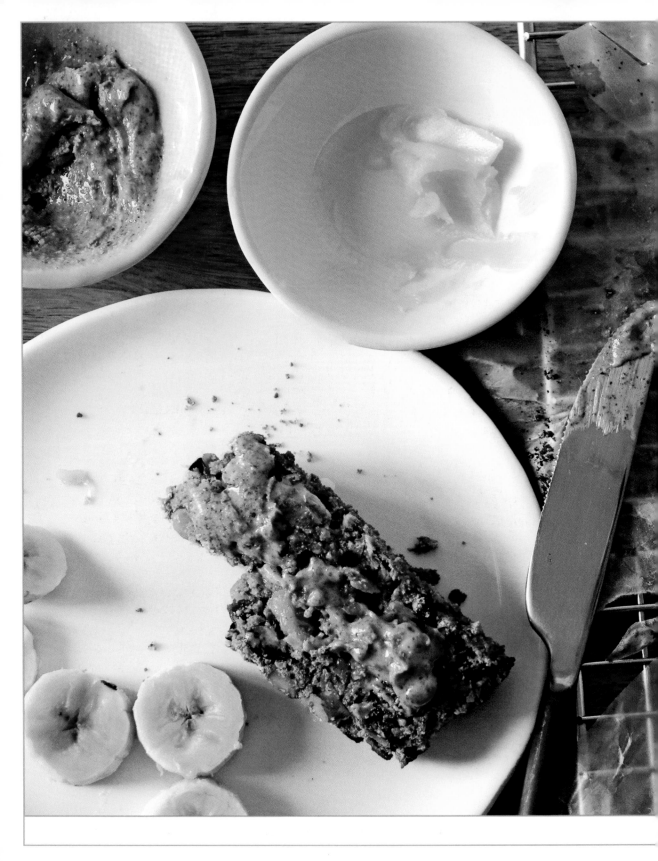

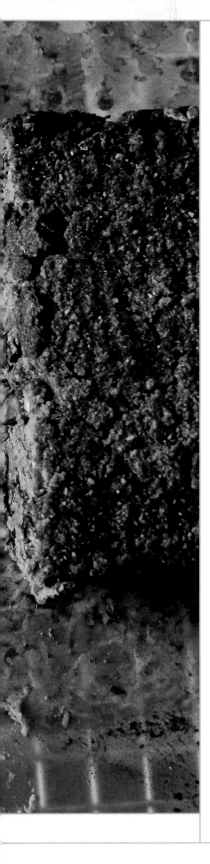

Banana Nut Bread

MAKES ONE LOAF; SERVES 10

2 large or 3 small ripe bananas, mashed

½ cup raisins

½ cup hulled pumpkin seeds

¼ cup hulled sunflower seeds

¼ cup chia seeds

½ cup chopped pecans

1 cup chopped walnuts

½ cup cocoa nibs

3 twists, or one pinch, of sea salt

4 large eggs

½ cup coconut flour

2 tablespoons honey

2 tablespoons pure maple syrup

2 teaspoons ground cinnamon

Coconut sugar

Preheat the oven to 375°F. Line a loaf pan with parchment paper. In a large bowl, combine the bananas, raisins, pumpkin seeds, sunflower seeds, chia seeds, pecans, walnuts, cocoa nibs, salt, eggs, coconut flour, honey, maple syrup, and cinnamon and mix well. Pour the batter into the prepared pan and tap the bottom of the pan sharply against the counter to remove any air bubbles. Sprinkle the top lightly with coconut sugar. Bake for 45 minutes, or until the top starts to brown. Let cool slightly in the pan before cutting. Top with ghee or a nut butter for a quick breakfast or satisfying snack.

Sweet Potato Toast

MAKES 4 TO 6 SLICES

**1 large sweet potato,
cut lengthwise into ¼-inch-thick slices**

Put the sweet potato slices in the toaster, turn
the time all the way up, and toast for two or three
cycles, or until the slices have a few brown bubbles
on them. Top with whatever you want! I have served
it both sweet, with Madagascar vanilla ghee,
almond butter, pear, and cinnamon; and savory,
with unflavored ghee, shredded slow-cooked beef,
avocado, and freshly cracked black pepper.

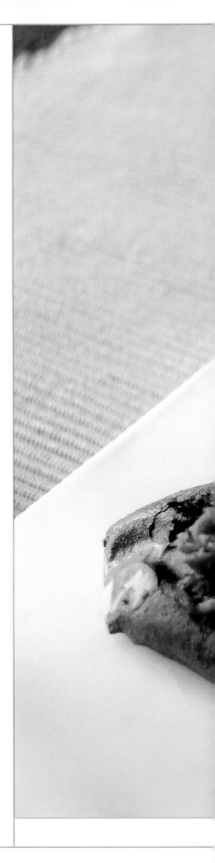

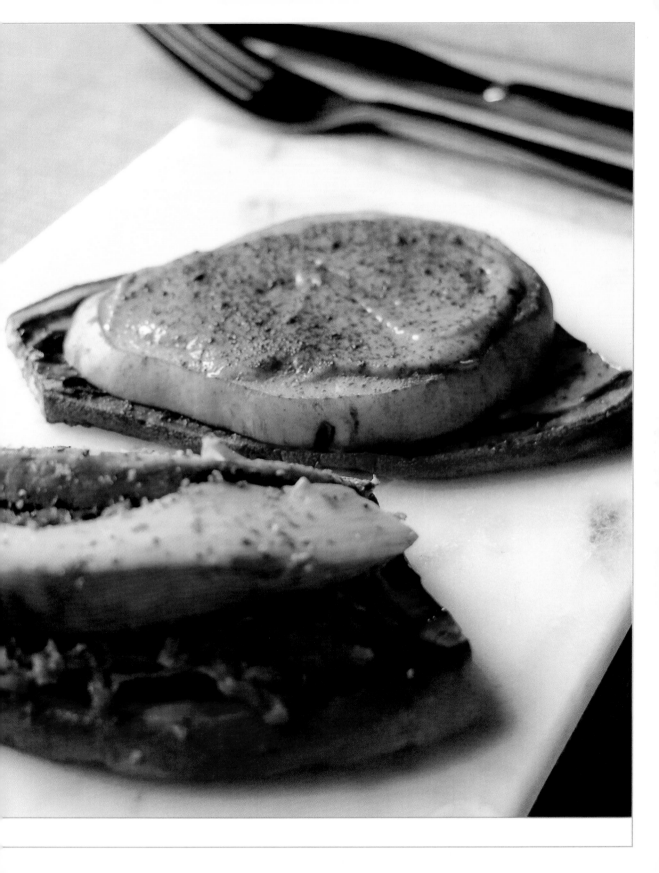

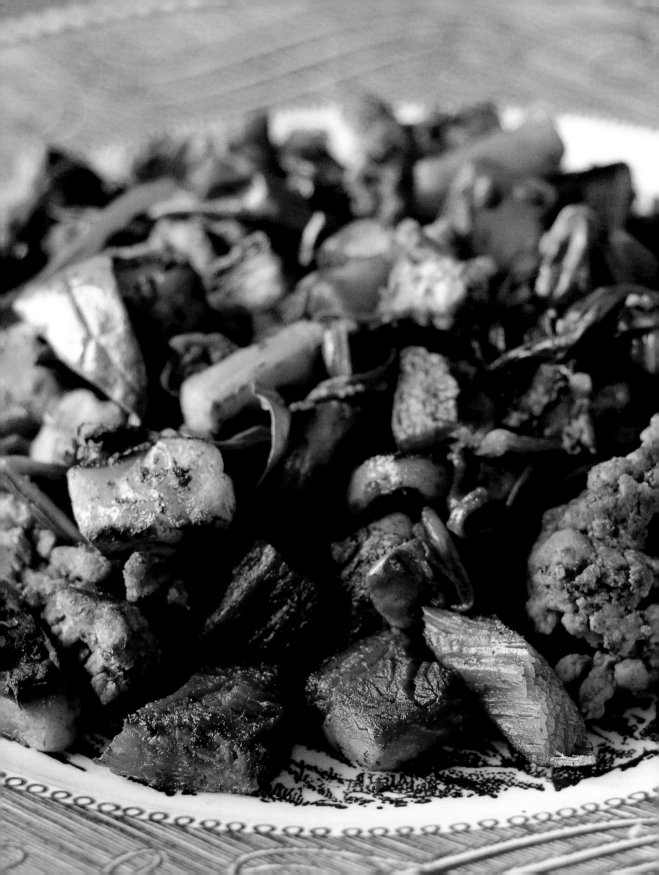

Butternut Squash Hash

SERVES 4

½ pound bacon

1 pound all-natural grass-fed ground beef

Sea salt and freshly ground black pepper

6 ounces fresh spinach

1 Roasted Butternut Squash (see page 270)

Heat a large sauté pan over medium heat, add the bacon, and cook, flipping a couple of times, until done the way you like it. Remove the bacon from the pan and set aside to cool; pour off the rendered bacon fat into a mason jar or heatproof container, leaving a coating of fat in the pan. Place the pan back over medium heat and add the ground beef; cook until there is no more pink and season with salt and pepper. While the beef cooks, crumble the bacon. Set the beef aside in a small bowl. Without cleaning the pan, add the spinach and cook, stirring, until fully wilted. Add the crumbled bacon, beef, and butternut squash to the pan and stir to combine. Serve yourself and guests, or just plate up your portion and have leftovers for easy reheating later in the week!

Winter Sweet Potato Hash

SERVES 4

1 tablespoon coconut oil

1 large sweet potato, unpeeled, diced

1 pound ground bison

Salt and freshly ground black pepper

6 ounces fresh spinach, kale, or chard

8 tablespoons pomegranate seeds

1 avocado, peeled and sliced

In a large saucepan, melt the coconut oil over medium heat, swirling to coat the pan. Add the sweet potato and cook until the sides turn brown. Heat another pan over medium heat. Add the bison and season with salt and pepper. Cook, stirring occasionally, until cooked through. Transfer the bison to a large bowl. In the same pan, cook the spinach until fully wilted. Add the spinach and sweet potato to the bowl with the bison and stir to combine. Divide the hash among four plates and top each with one quarter of the pomegranate seeds and one quarter of the avocado.

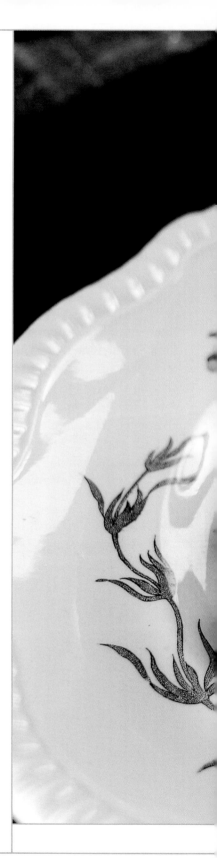

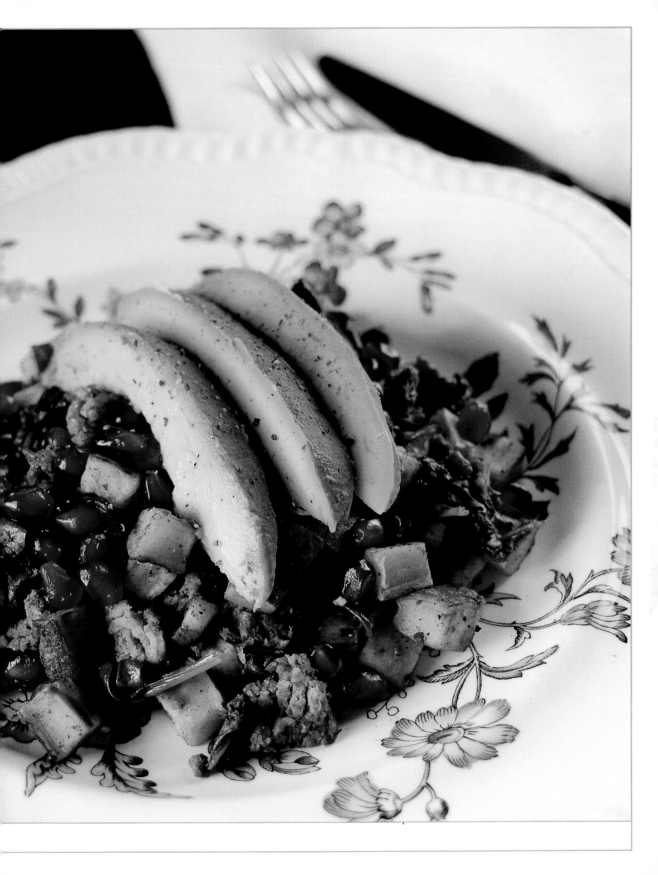

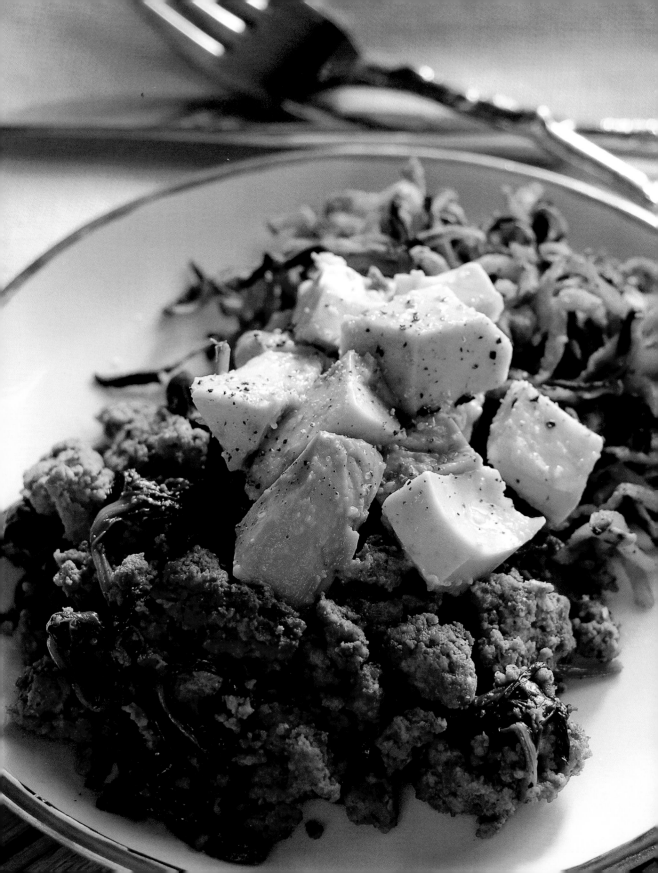

Easy Breakfast Hash

SERVES 1

1 tablespoon coconut oil (if using sweet potato) or ghee (for white potato) (see page 183)

½ sweet potato or white potato, shredded and excess water squeezed out

Salt

¼ pound all-natural, grass-fed ground beef

Freshly ground black pepper

2 handfuls of fresh spinach

¼ avocado, peeled

In a large sauté pan, melt the coconut oil over medium-high heat, swirling to coat the pan. Add the sweet potato and cook, stirring, until crispy and browned. Season lightly with salt. While the potato cooks, heat a second pan over medium heat and cook the ground beef all the way through, seasoning with salt and pepper. Toss the spinach in with the beef and stir frequently until it has wilted. Serve beef and sweet potato hash side by side on breakfast plate, and top with avocado.

Potato Crust Egg Bake

SERVES 8

2 medium sweet potatoes, peeled and shredded, excess water squeezed out

2 tablespoons ghee, melted

1 bunch kale, chopped

12 large eggs

½ teaspoons sea salt

½ teaspoons freshly ground black pepper

1 large tomato, thinly sliced

3 ounces cheese (I use almond milk cheese), shredded

Preheat the oven to 400°F. Combine the sweet potatoes and ghee in a large bowl. Transfer the potato to a cast-iron skillet or baking dish and begin to pack it down and up the sides of the dish to form a bowl shape. In a large bowl, combine the kale, eggs, salt, and pepper. Mix well and pour into the baking dish. Top with the tomato slices and pat dry with paper towels evenly across the top. Top with the cheese of your choice. Bake for 50 minutes, or until cooked in the middle.

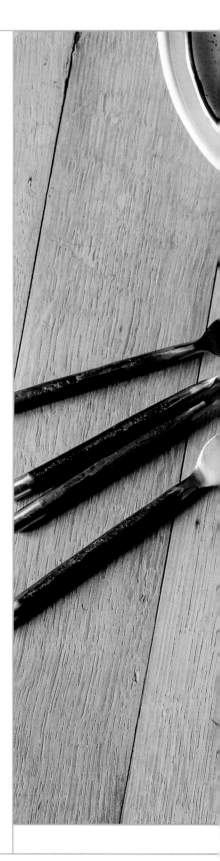

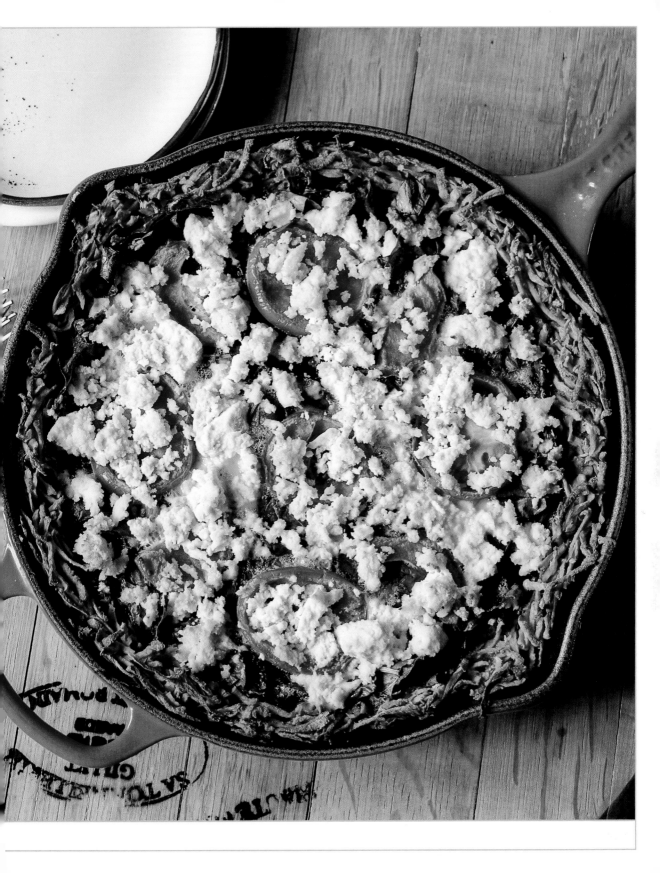

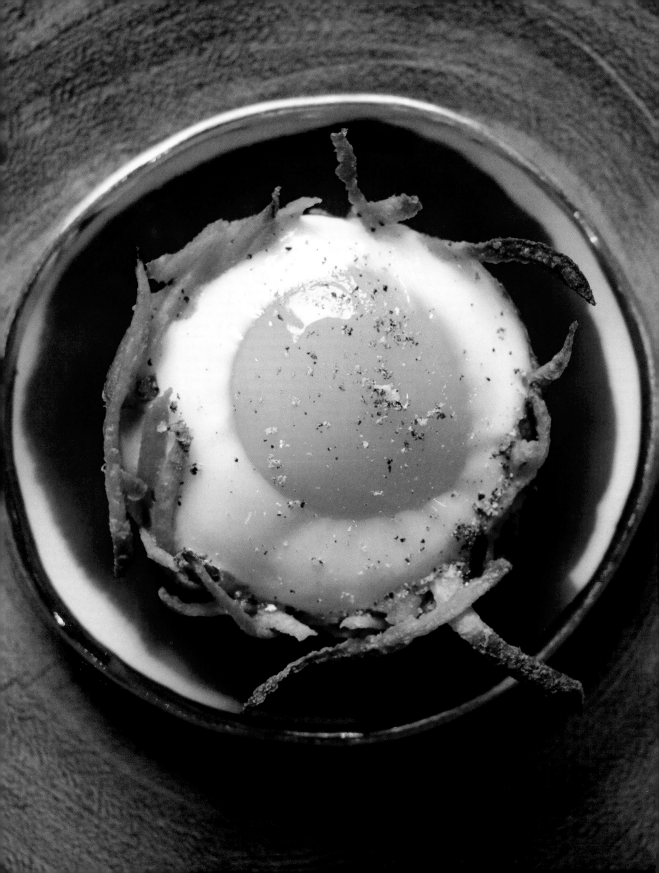

Breakfast Nest

SERVES 6

Coconut oil spray

2 tablespoons ghee (see page 183), melted

1 large sweet potato, shredded

12 large eggs

Salt and freshly ground black pepper

Preheat the oven to 350°F. Use the coconut oil spray to grease a 12-cup muffin tin. In a medium bowl, combine the ghee and sweet potato and toss to combine. Evenly distribute the potato among the prepared muffin cups. Pack down the potato with your hands or with the bottom of a small cup to form a nest. Crack an egg into each hole and bake for 35 to 40 minutes, or until the whites are cooked. Season with salt and pepper.

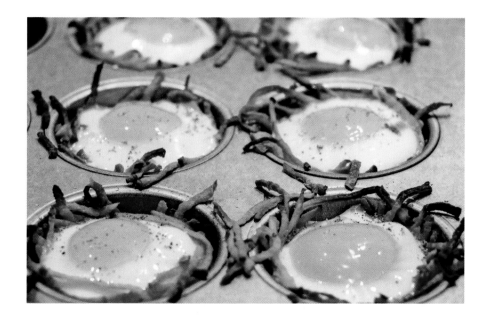

Breakfast Tacos

SERVES 2

4 bacon slices

4 corn tortillas

4 large eggs

¼ cup cheese or ½ mashed avocado

Salt and freshly ground black pepper

Put the bacon in a skillet, then set the skillet over medium heat. (This will keep the bacon flat instead of curling.) Cook until the bacon is to your liking, then transfer to paper towels and roll up. Keep the bacon fat in the pan. In a second, larger pan, warm the tortillas over medium heat, overlapping them as little as possible. In the meantime, scramble the eggs in the pan with the bacon fat. Flip the tortillas and add the cheese of your choice on top. You can also skip the cheese and put avocado on top at the end. When the eggs are done, evenly distribute them among the tortillas. Once the bottom of the tortillas are a little brown, remove from the pan and top with salt, pepper, and a slice of avocado if you like. Top with the bacon and serve.

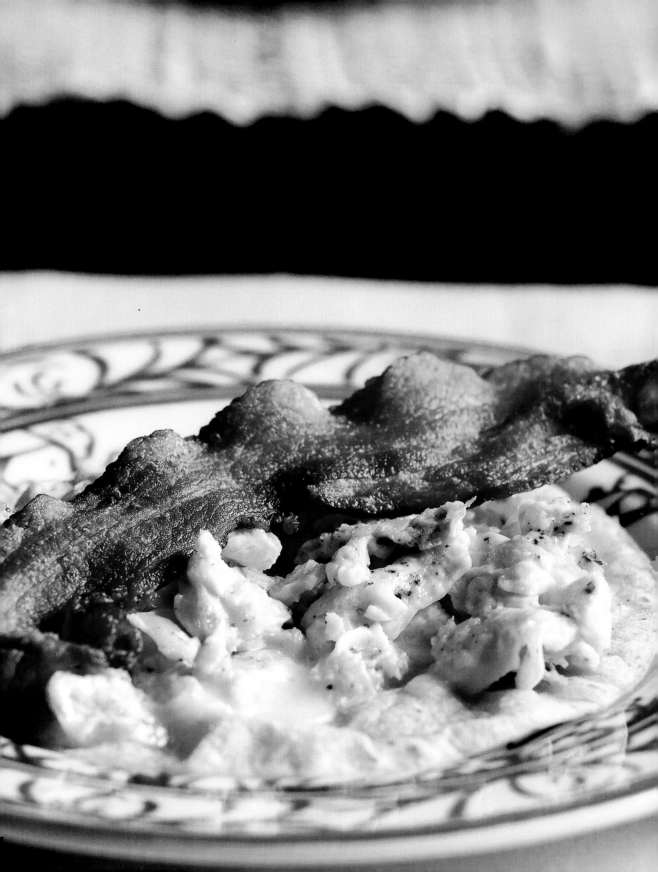

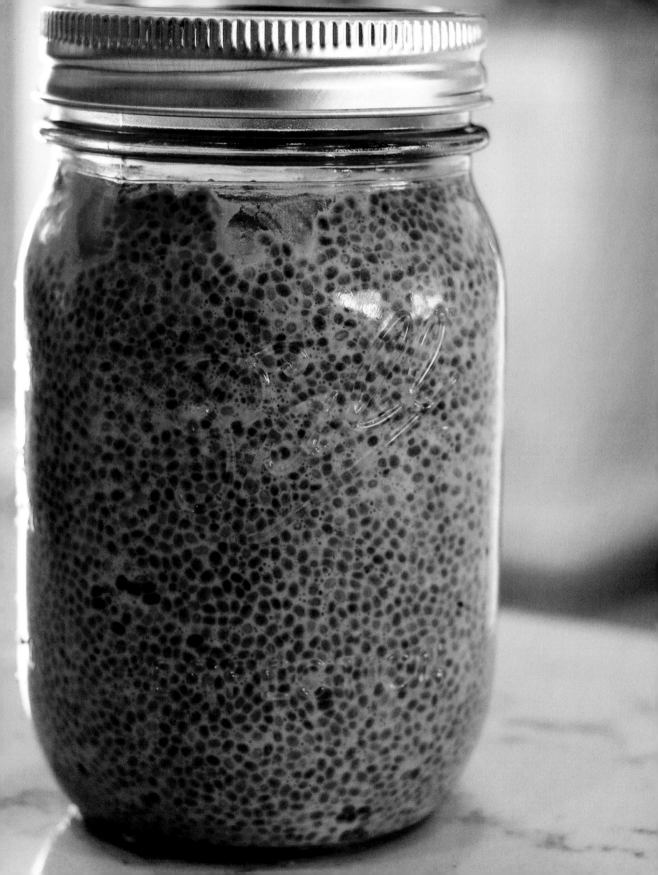

Chia Pudding

SERVES 4

½ cup chia seeds

1½ cups almond milk, or 1 (14-ounce) can lite coconut milk

Combine the chia seeds and almond milk in a bowl. Stir the seeds a few times for 5 minutes, then store in the fridge. The pudding will be ready to eat after about 20 minutes, but will keep in the refrigerator for up to 1 week.

Easy Berry Chia Pudding

SERVES 1

½ cup Chia Pudding (see page 225)

2 tablespoons hemp seeds

½ cup fresh berries of your choice

Maple Syrup Coconut Flakes (see page 297)

Put the presoaked chia pudding in a bowl and top with the hemp seeds, berries, and coconut flakes.

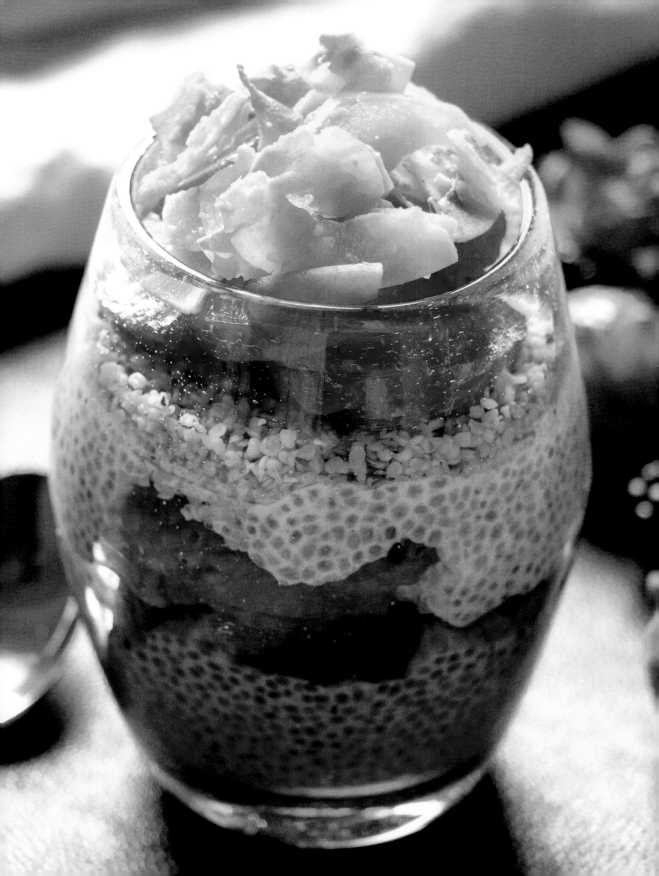

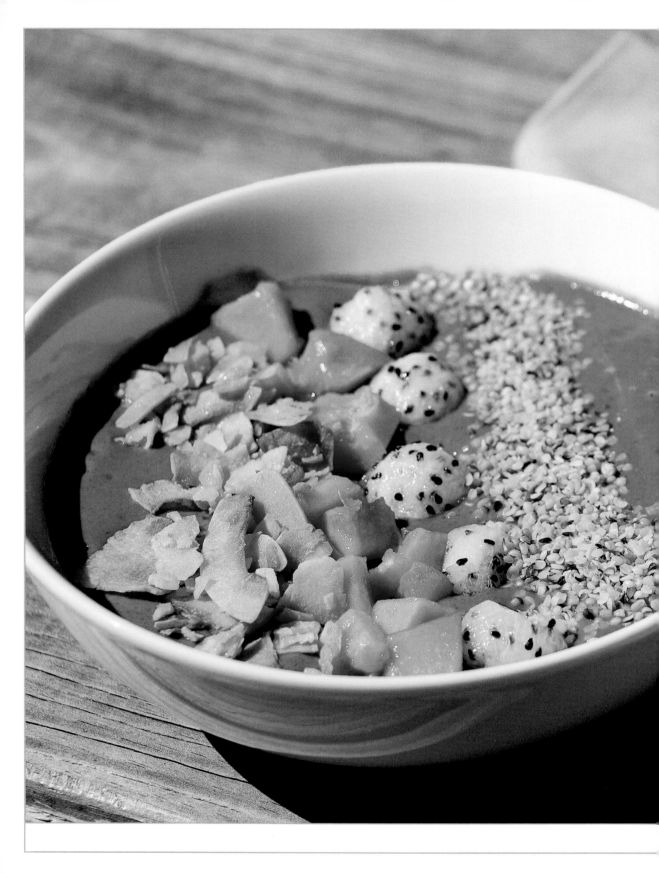

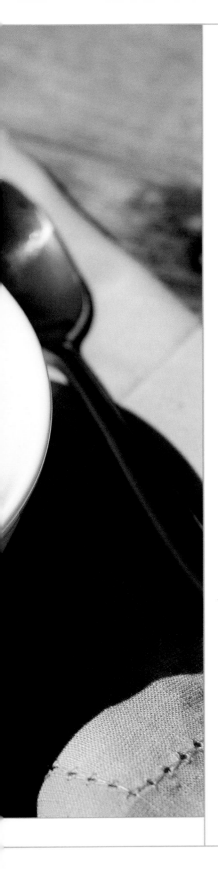

Super-Duper Green Smoothie Bowl

SERVES 1

½ frozen banana

½ cup frozen cauliflower

2 big handfuls fresh spinach

1 teaspoon chlorella

1 teaspoon honey

1 tablespoon cashew butter

1 tablespoon hemp seeds

½ cup dragon fruit

¼ cup papaya

2 tablespoons Maple Syrup Coconut Flakes (see page 297)

Combine the banana, cauliflower, spinach, chlorella, honey, and cashew butter in a blender. Start the blender and add water slowly until you reach the desired thickness. Pour the smoothie into a bowl and top with the hemp seeds, dragon fruit, papaya, and coconut flakes. Banana, mulberries, or a grain-free/gluten-free granola would also go well on top.

Green Smoothie

SERVES 1

2 large handfuls fresh spinach

⅓ apple, cored

⅓ lemon, peeled and seeded

½ banana, frozen

¼ avocado, peeled (optional)

Combine the spinach, apple, lemon, banana, and avocado, if using, in a blender and blend until smooth. Add water as needed to reach the desired consistency.

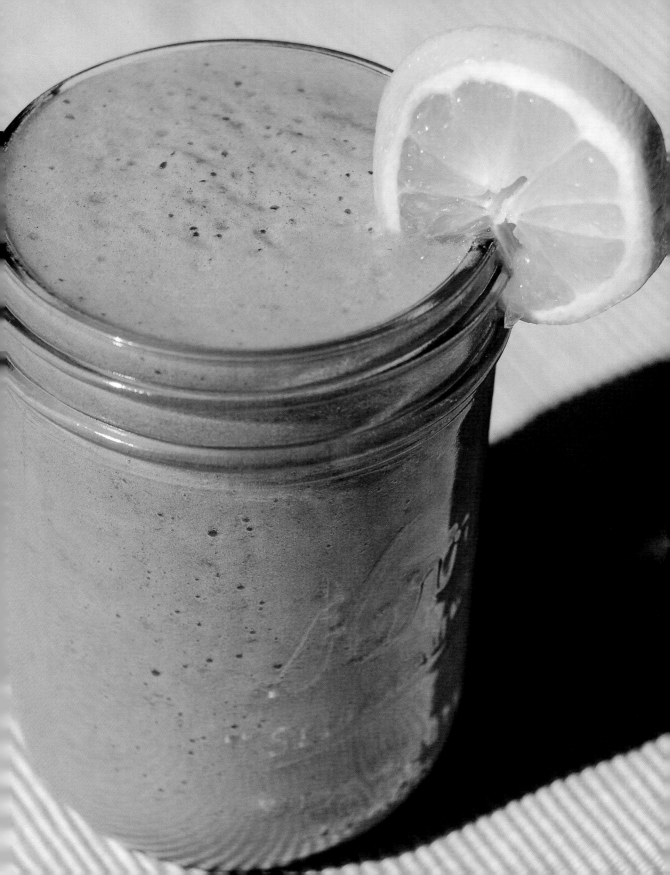

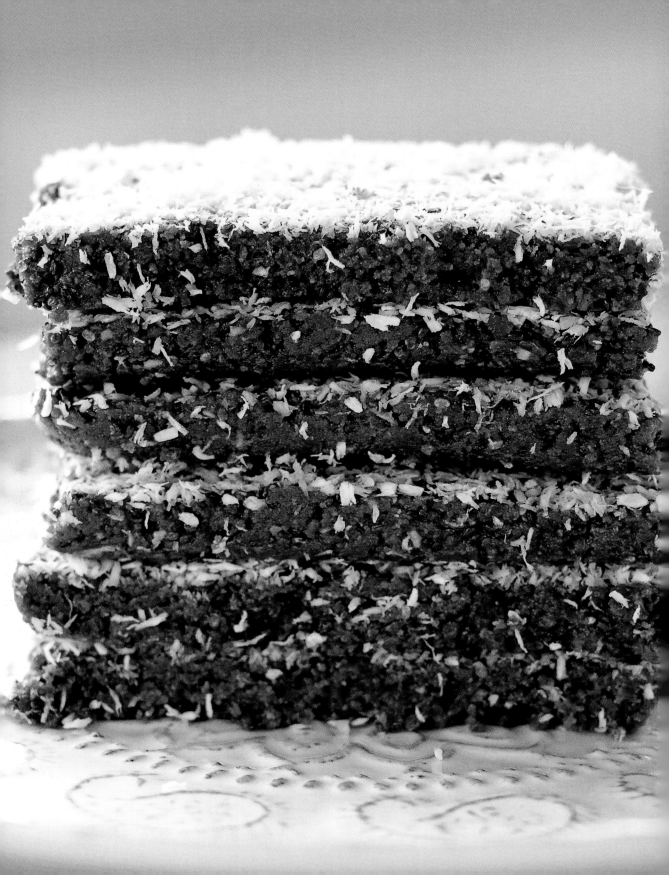

Raw Super Bars

MAKES 24 BARS

12 pitted dates

⅓ cup chia seeds

1 tablespoon manuka honey

1 tablespoon honey

⅔ cup almond butter

⅓ cup hemp seeds

2 teaspoons ashwagandha powder (optional)

2 teaspoons cordyceps powder (optional)

4 teaspoons maca powder

2 scoops protein powder (optional)

2 tablespoons brain octane oil, MCT oil, or coconut oil

2 teaspoons ground cinnamon

⅔ cup goji berries

½ cup cocoa nibs

Pinch of sea salt

Reduced-fat finely shredded coconut

Combine the dates, chia seeds, honeys, almond butter, hemp seeds, ashwagandha, cordyceps, if using, maca, protein powder, brain octane oil, cinnamon, goji berries, cocoa nibs, and sea salt in a food processor. Process well. Transfer to a rimmed baking sheet and pack the mixture down very well. Sprinkle shredded coconut over the top to cover completely. Shift the pan side to side to help cover evenly. Refrigerate for about 1 hour to set before you cut into bars. Store in the fridge in an airtight container.

Grain-Free Granola

SERVES 10 TO 12

1 cup unsweetened coconut flakes

1 cup almonds, sliced

½ cup pecans, chopped

½ cup hulled pumpkin seeds

½ cup hulled sunflower seeds

½ cup raisins

⅓ cup chia seeds

⅓ cup hemp seeds

2 tablespoons coconut oil

1 teaspoon ground cinnamon

1 teaspoon pure vanilla extract

3 tablespoons honey

¼ teaspoon sea salt

Preheat the oven to 350ºF. Combine the coconut flakes, almonds, pecans, pumpkin seeds, sunflower seeds, raisins, chia seeds, hemp seeds, coconut oil, cinnamon, vanilla, honey, and salt in a large bowl, and then spread the mixture over a rimmed baking sheet. Bake for 20 minutes, or until the edges start to brown. Let cool completely before you store (in an airtight container) to help the chunks of granola form.

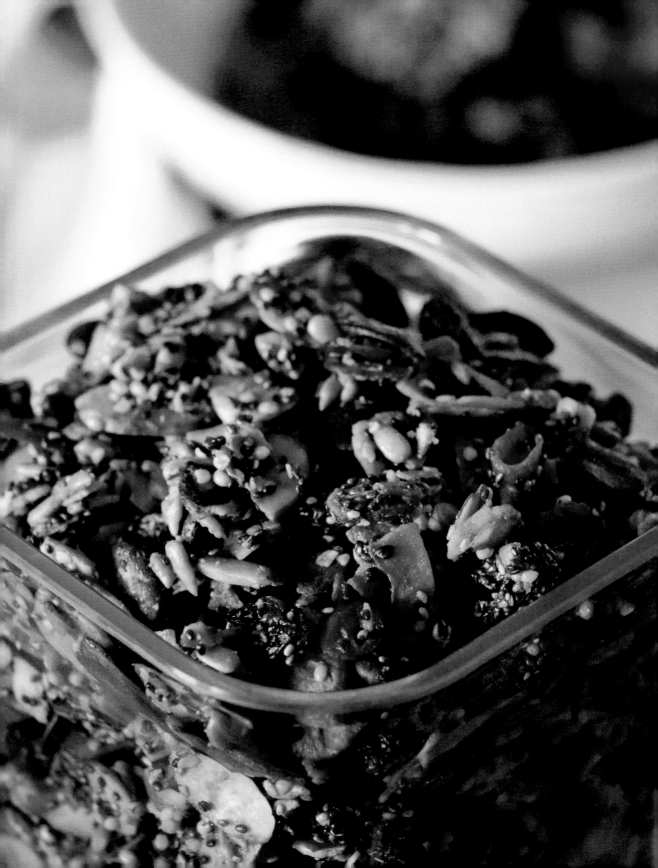

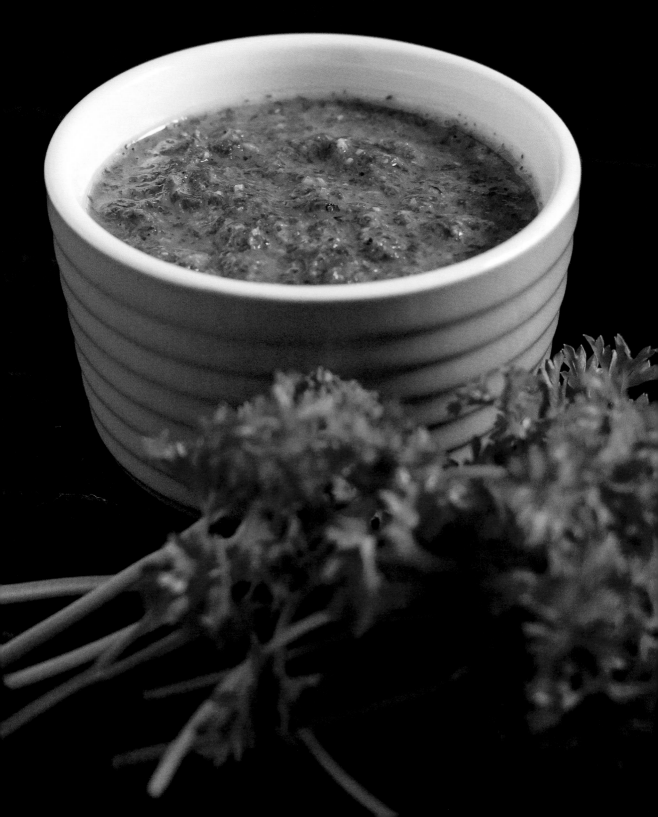

Chimichurri

SERVES 8 TO 12

1 bunch fresh parsley

3 garlic cloves

¼ cup olive oil

1 tablespoon apple cider vinegar

1 teaspoon coconut vinegar

Juice of ½ lemon

½ teaspoon freshly ground black pepper

¾ teaspoon sea salt

½ teaspoon dried oregano

½ teaspoon dried basil

¾ teaspoon chipotle chile flakes

1 tablespoon chopped fresh onion

1 teaspoon honey

Combine the parsley, garlic, olive oil, vinegars, lemon juice, pepper, salt, oregano, basil, chile flakes, onion, and honey in a food processor and process until smooth. Serve with beef, pork, or vegetables. Store in the fridge for up to 5 days.

Sauces, Dressings, and Dairy Substitutes

While some of these are available in store-bought versions, you'll never get quite the same fresh flavor as homemade. Make them a day or two ahead of time and bring to room temperature before adding to your next creation.

Cashew Cheese

SERVES 6 TO 8

1 cup raw cashews

1 tablespoon apple cider vinegar

1 tablespoon fresh lemon juice

3 tablespoons nutritional yeast

2 tablespoons olive oil

2 tablespoons hulled sunflower seeds

1 teaspoon sea salt

1 teaspoon dried rosemary

¼ teaspoon freshly cracked black pepper

2 teaspoons honey

Combine the cashews, vinegar, lemon juice, nutritional yeast, olive oil, sunflower seeds, salt, rosemary, pepper, and honey in a food processor and process until smooth. Serve on salads in place of dairy-based cheese. Store in the fridge for up to 5 days.

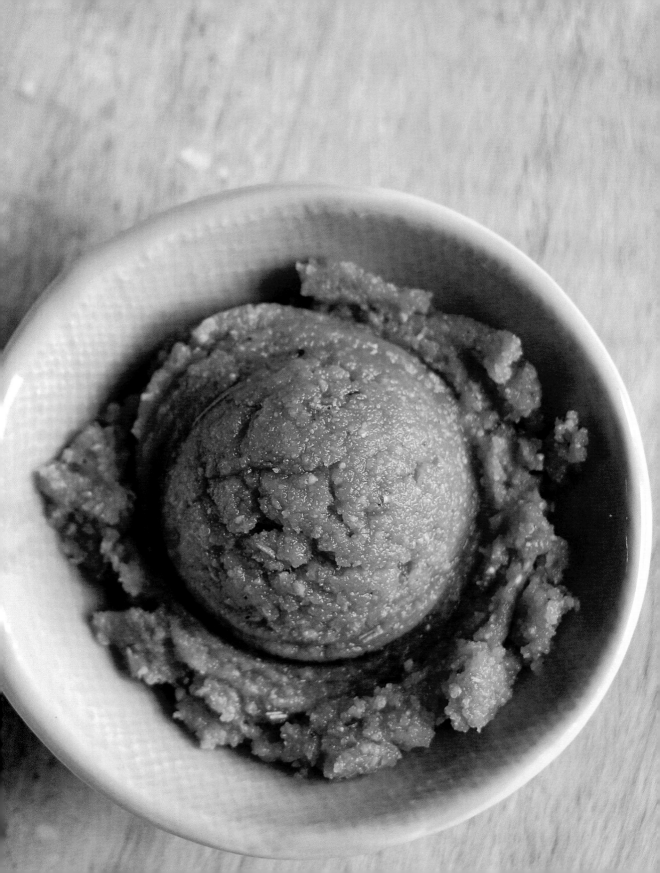

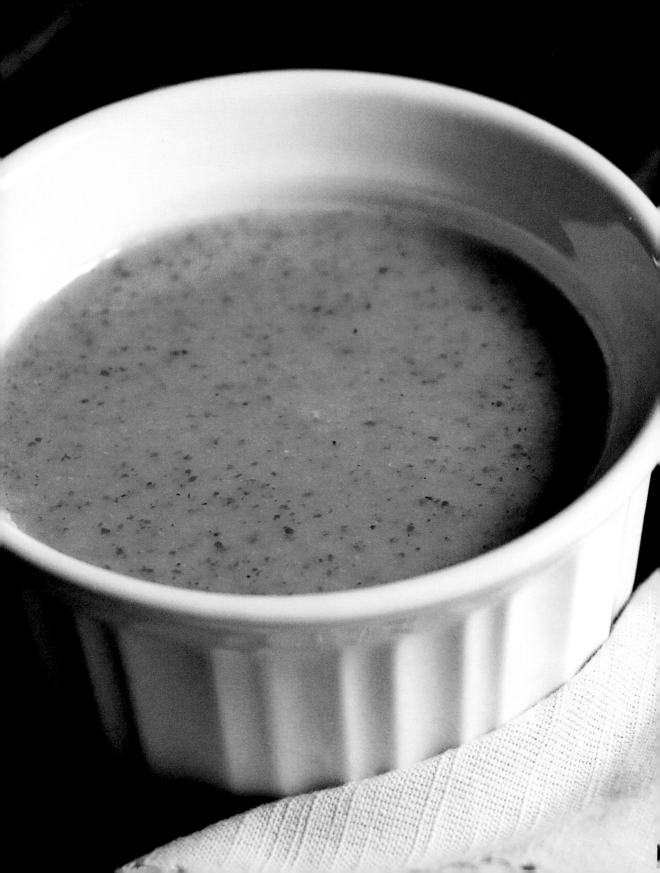

Honey Mustard

SERVES 6 TO 8 (1 TABLESPOON PER SERVING)

¼ cup olive oil

1 tablespoon apple cider vinegar

2 tablespoons honey

3 tablespoons stone-ground mustard

1 tablespoon fresh lemon juice

Sea salt and freshly ground black pepper

Whisk together the olive oil, vinegar, honey, mustard, lemon juice, 2 tablespoons water, and salt and pepper to taste in a small bowl, or combine in a mason jar, seal, and shake. Will keep in the fridge for months.

Classic Balsamic Vinaigrette

SERVES 6 TO 8

¼ cup olive oil

2 tablespoons balsamic glaze

1 tablespoon balsamic vinegar

1 tablespoon fresh lemon juice

¼ teaspoon sea salt

¼ teaspoon freshly ground black pepper

Whisk together the olive oil, balsamic glaze, balsamic vinegar, lemon juice, salt, and pepper in a bowl, or combine in a mason jar, seal, and shake. Will keep in the fridge for months.

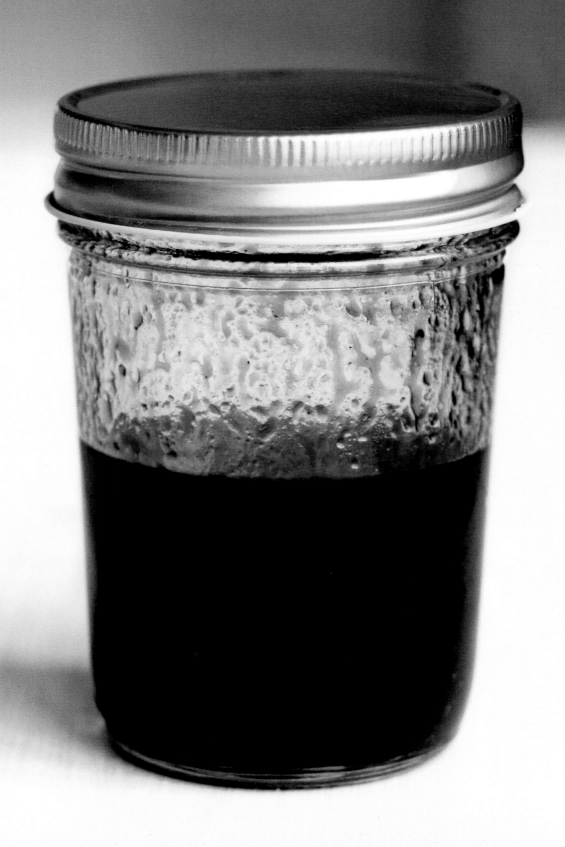

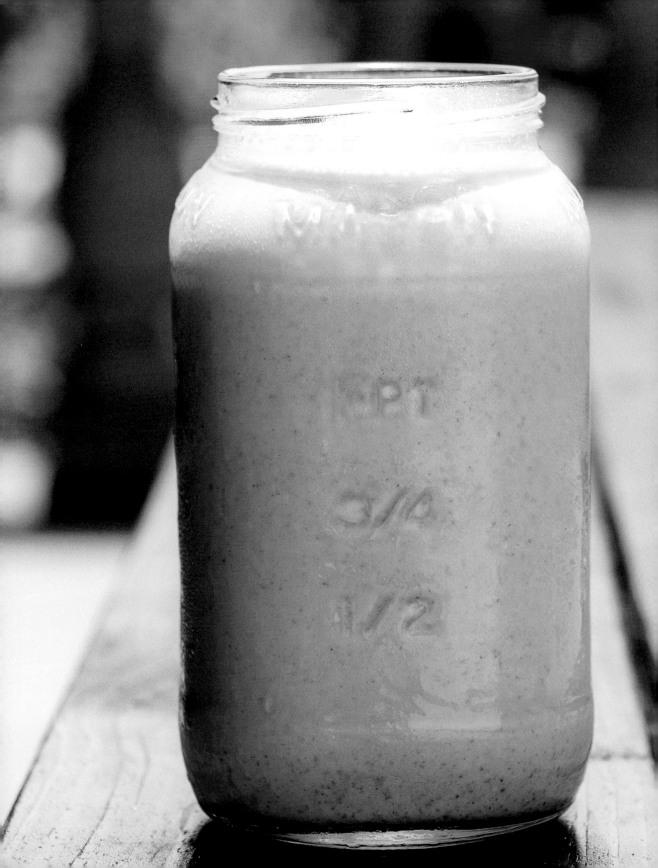

Almond Milk

SERVES 6

2 cups raw almonds

3 pitted dates

¼ teaspoon ground cinnamon

Pinch of sea salt

Cheesecloth

Put the almonds in a bowl and add enough water to completely cover them. Soak overnight. The next day, drain the almonds and transfer them to a blender along with the dates, cinnamon, sea salt, and 6 cups filtered water. Blend on high for about 1 minute. Place a layer of cheesecloth over a large bowl and carefully pour the unfiltered milk into the bowl; lift the cheesecloth and wait for the milk to strain out, lightly squeezing the almond pulp to extract all the liquid. Transfer to a mason jar or sealed container and store in the fridge for up to 1 week.

Simple Slow-Cooker Beef

SERVES 8 TO 10

1 tablespoon olive oil	2 teaspoons dried rosemary
1 teaspoon sea salt	4 pounds beef (any large cut; I used two 2-pound roasts)
1 teaspoon freshly ground black pepper	
1 teaspoon onion powder	Fresh rosemary, chopped
1 teaspoon garlic powder	Fresh thyme

Rub the olive oil, salt, pepper, onion powder, garlic powder, and dried rosemary into the meat. Put the meat in the slow cooker, cover, and cook on High for 1 hour, then turn the heat to Low and cook for 6 hours more. Shred the meat in the slow cooker and allow it to reabsorb all the juices. Serve with fresh rosemary and thyme.

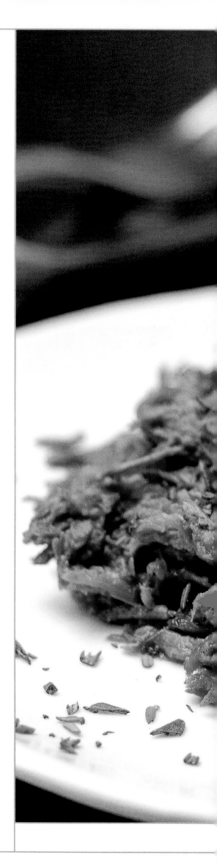

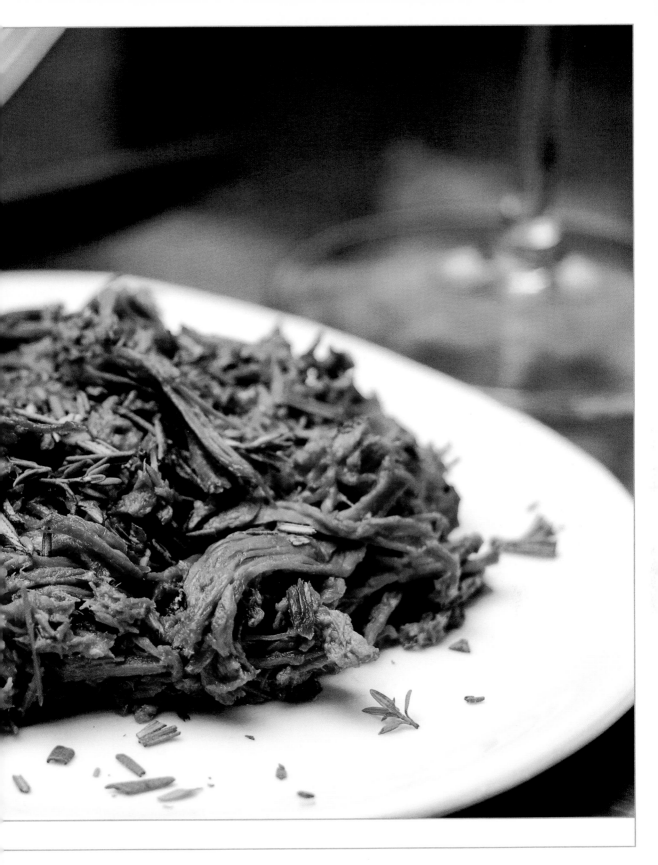

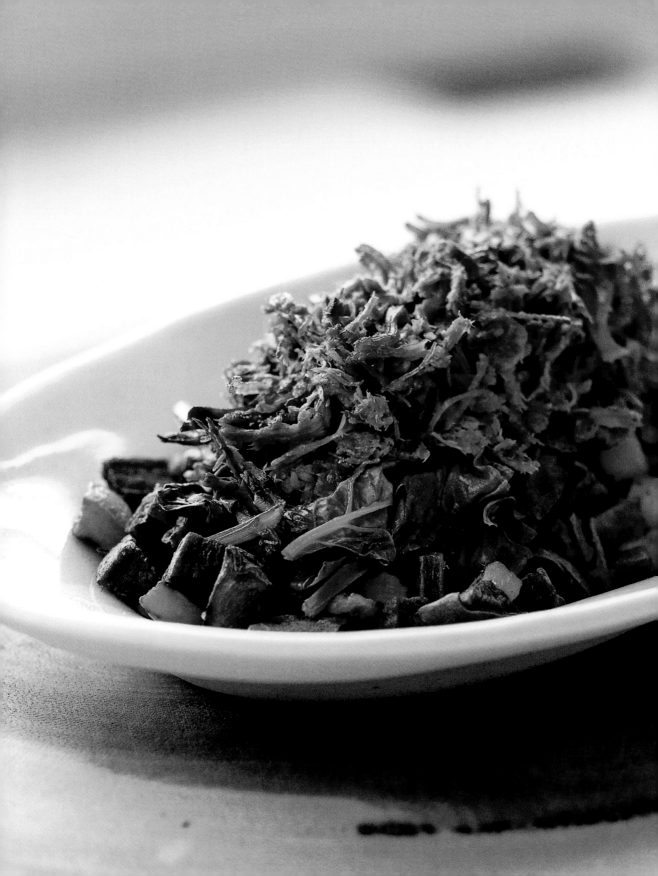

Harvest Dinner

SERVES 4

2 tablespoons olive oil

4 to 6 carrots, diced

2 purple sweet potatoes, cubed

Sea salt

2 teaspoons ghee

6 ounces fresh spinach

2 heaping cups Simple Slow-Cooker Beef (see page 246)

Heat the oil in a skillet over medium heat. Add the carrots and potatoes and cook, stirring, until slightly browned, adding the salt halfway through. Heat a separate pan over medium heat. Melt the ghee, then cook the spinach, stirring, until fully wilted. Divide the potatoes, carrots, and spinach evenly among four plates and top each with ½ cup of the beef.

Spaghetti and Meatballs

SERVES 6

SPAGHETTI

2 spaghetti squashes, halved and seeded

Olive oil

MEATBALLS

1 pound ground bison (also called buffalo)

1 pound ground beef (85% lean)

2 teaspoons white wine vinegar

1 large egg

1 tablespoon freshly ground black pepper

1 tablespoon sea salt

1 teaspoon onion powder

1 teaspoon garlic powder

SAUCE

5 small to medium tomatoes, chopped

1 (6-ounce) can tomato paste

1 teaspoon dried basil

1 teaspoon sea salt

1 teaspoon freshly ground black pepper

1 teaspoon dried oregano

¼ cup olive oil

Fresh basil

Make the spaghetti squash: Preheat the oven to 425°F. Rub each spaghetti squash half with a little olive oil and place on a baking sheet. Roast for 45 minutes, or until you can poke them with a fork and they are soft.

Make the meatballs: In a large bowl, combine the bison, beef, vinegar, egg, pepper, salt, onion powder, and garlic powder. Work the mixture together with your hands to combine. Wash your hands. Heat a large pan over medium heat. (No need to spray anything in the pan—the meat has plenty of fat.) Using your hands, form the meat mixture into balls and transfer them straight into the pan. Work fast. By the time you fill the pan, you will be ready to start flipping. I like to flip them on at least four sides. You may have to cook them in two batches.

Make the sauce: Put the tomatoes in a medium saucepan set over medium-low heat. Add the tomato paste, dried basil, salt, pepper, oregano, olive oil, and ½ cup water. Simmer and cook down a little, stirring regularly, for about 10 minutes. Place a fist-sized serving of squash on each plate, then top with 2 tablespoons of sauce, 2 meatballs, and fresh basil.

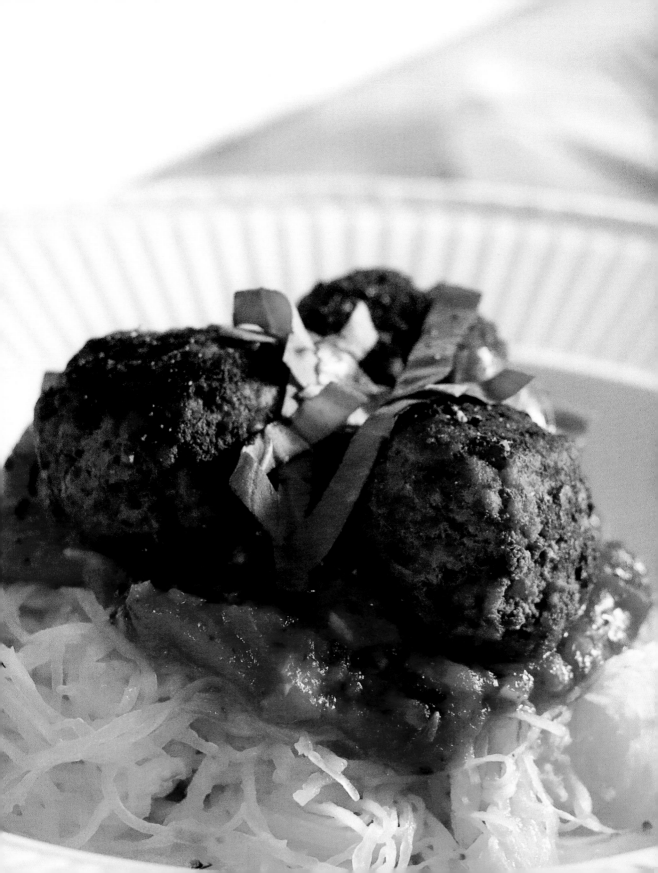

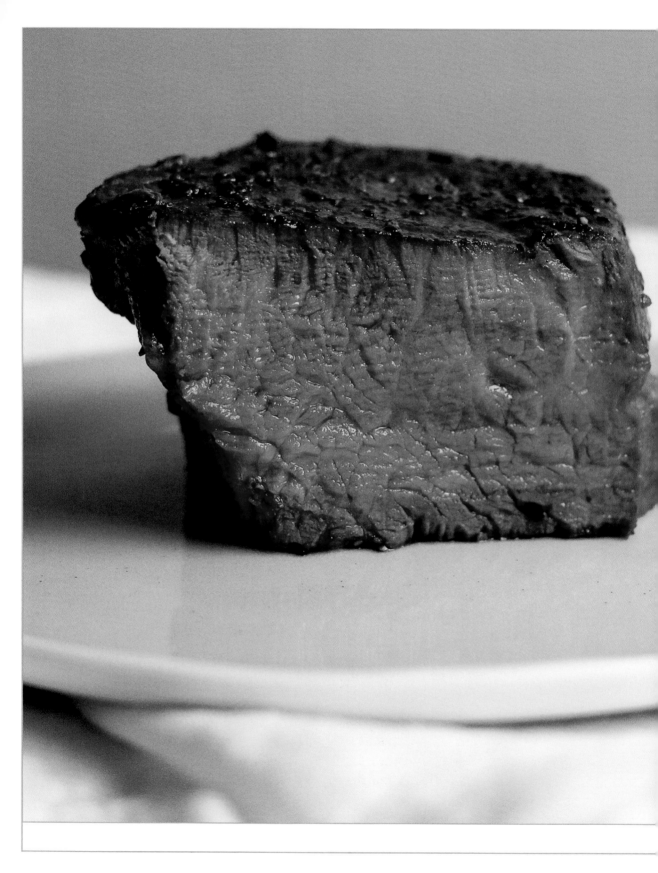

Perfect Grilled Steak

SERVES AS MANY AS YOU LIKE

| Steaks | Sea salt and freshly ground black pepper |

Remove the steak from the fridge at least 30 minutes and up to 2 hours before cooking to allow them to come to room temperature; flip and move them around the counter so they don't sit in the same cold spot. (Warming the steaks up first allows you to cook them on a high temperature for a short amount of time. This helps you achieve hard sear marks, giving the meat caramelized flavor without having to leave it on the grill for too long, which will make the meat tough.) Heat your grill to 400 to 450°F. Season the steaks well with salt and pepper. Once the grill is ready, put your steaks on. When the first side has good black grill marks, flip the steaks over. When the second side has grill marks, flip them one more time, turning them 45 degrees to form those beautiful #hashtag markings. If they still need more time, you can flip them to the second side again, rotating them 45 degrees. It's impossible to give a cooking time for steak. You need to get good at poking your meat with the tongs to tell how done it is. (See my notes in chapter 15.) This goes for all meat. If it is really squishy, it's not even close. If it is very firm, it's overdone. You want the meat to squish just a little; that is your medium.

Pulled Pork

SERVES 8 TO 10

4 pounds pork
(any large cut)

2 tablespoons olive oil

1 tablespoon sea salt

1 tablespoon freshly
ground black pepper

2 teaspoons
mustard powder

2 teaspoons
onion powder

2 teaspoons
garlic powder

2 teaspoons
chili powder

2 teaspoons paprika

Rub the meat with the olive oil. Mix the salt, pepper, mustard powder, onion powder, garlic powder, chili powder, and paprika in a small bowl with a fork. Rub the seasoning on all sides of the pork and put it in the slow cooker. Cover and cook on High for the first hour, then turn the heat to Low and let it cook anywhere between 6 and 9 hours. Flip the meat about halfway through. When it is finished, shred the meat in the slow cooker so it can absorb all the juices.

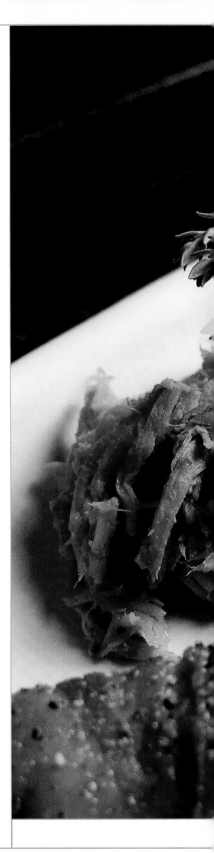

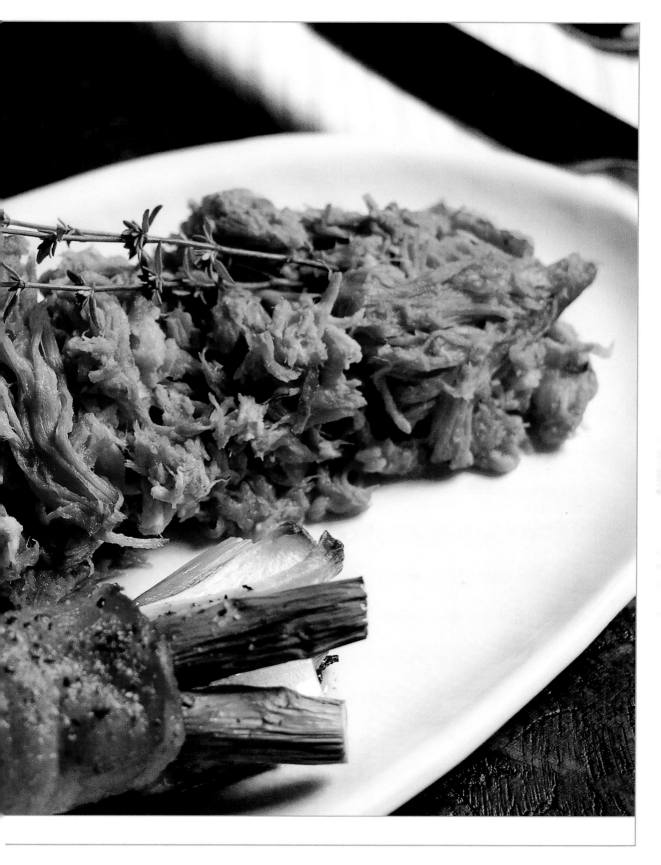

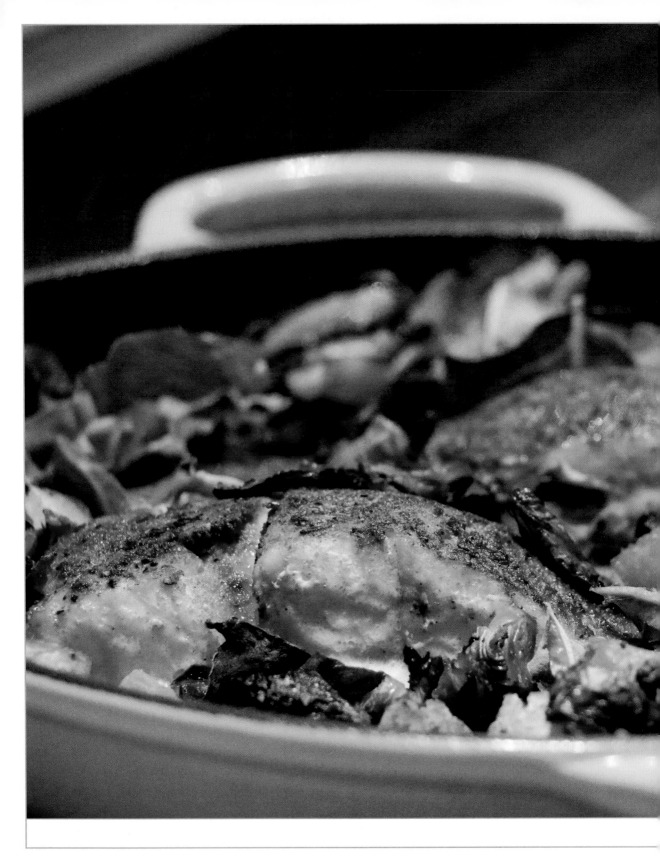

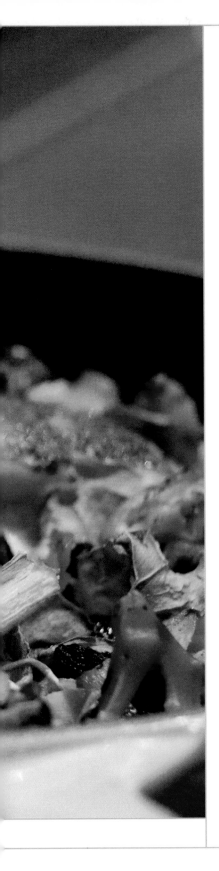

Salmon Skillet Dinner

SERVES 2

12 ounces salmon, cut into two 6-ounce portions

Sea salt and freshly ground black pepper to taste

¼ teaspoon ground turmeric

¼ teaspoon curry powder

¼ teaspoon ground ginger

1 teaspoon ghee

1 cup leftover vegetables (optional)

10 to 12 cherry tomatoes, halved

4 to 6 chard leaves, chopped

Take the salmon out of the fridge and let it warm up on the counter for at least 30 minutes. Preheat the oven to 350°F. Heat a cast-iron skillet over medium-high heat. Season the salmon with the salt, pepper, turmeric, curry powder, and ginger. Once the pan is hot, add the ghee and let it melt, then put the salmon skin-side up in the pan. Once the salmon begins to lift off the pan or the top is brown, flip it over. Add the leftover vegetables, if using, and chard to the pan and arrange around the salmon, with the tomatoes on top. Bake for about 15 minutes, or until you see white starting to come out of the salmon. When you take the salmon out of the pan, the skin should stick and stay in the pan; it will lift off when it cools. Portion out the vegetables onto each plate along with the salmon.

Grilled Chicken Legs

SERVES 2

4 chicken legs

Sea salt and freshly ground black pepper

Herbes de Provence

Take the chicken legs out of the fridge and let them warm up on the counter for at least 30 minutes. Preheat the oven to 350°F. Heat a grill pan over medium-high heat. Season the chicken legs with salt, pepper, and herbes de Provence. Add the chicken legs to the skillet—they should sizzle when they hit the pan. Cook on the first side long enough to make sear marks and until the legs lift off the pan easily. Flip them over and finish them off in the oven for about 15 minutes or until they are cooked through.

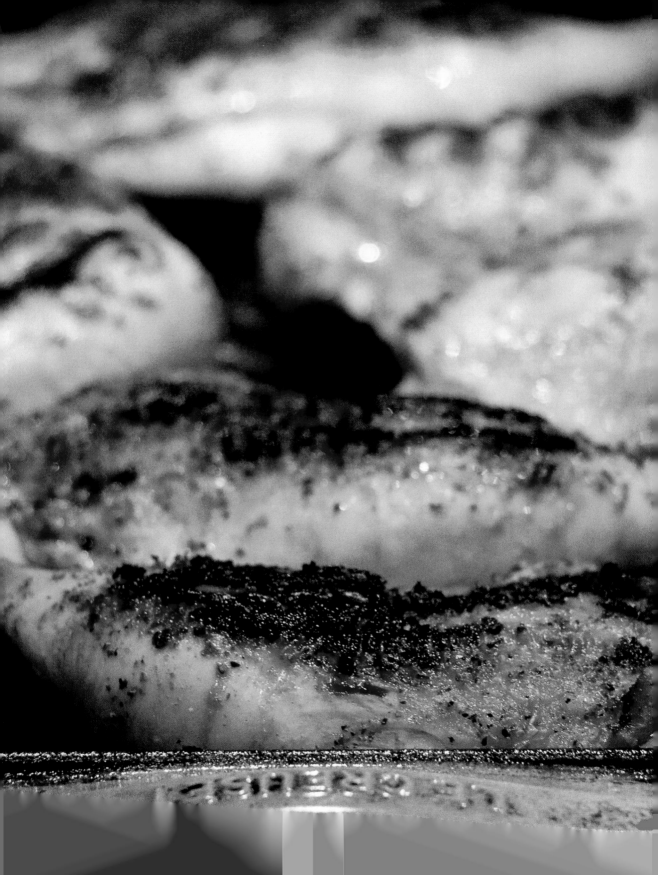

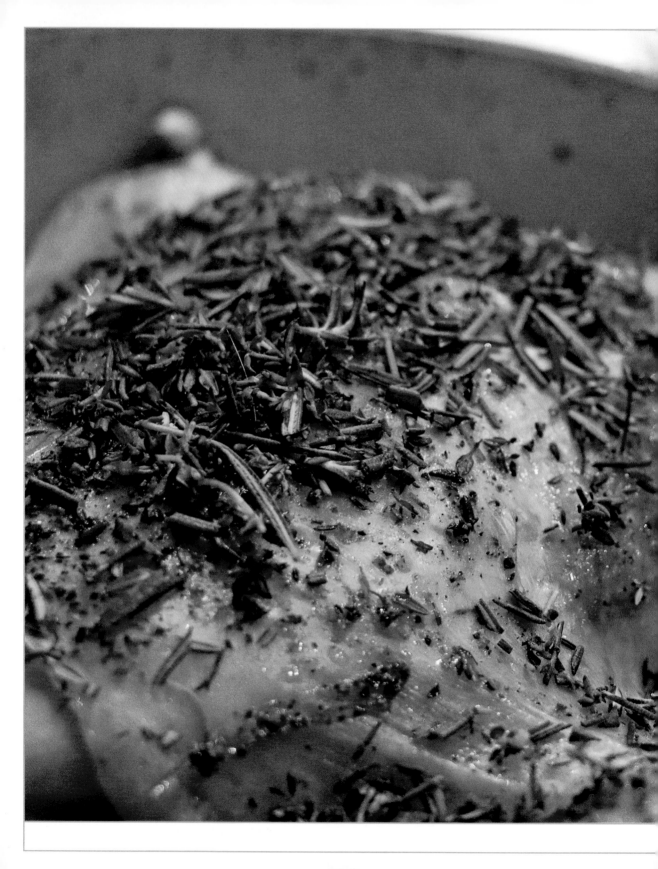

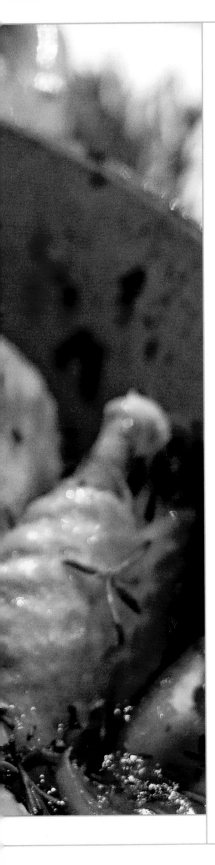

Lemon Chicken

SERVES 4 TO 6

1 (4- to 6-pound) whole chicken

Olive oil

Sea salt and freshly ground black pepper

2 medium sweet yellow onions, chopped

1 lemon, cut into 6 wedges

Fresh rosemary

Fresh thyme

Remove the chicken from the fridge and let it sit out for at least 30 minutes. Preheat the oven to 375°F. Rub the chicken with olive oil and season with salt and pepper. Place the chicken in a Dutch oven (or an oven-safe pot with a lid). Spread the onions and lemon wedges around the chicken in the pot. Place in the oven, covered, and bake for about 90 minutes, or until the skin is crispy and a meat thermometer reads 165°F when inserted into the thickest part of the chicken. Garnish with fresh rosemary and thyme.

Summer Chicken Salad

SERVES 4

2 pounds skinless, boneless chicken thighs

Sea salt and freshly ground black pepper

1 pineapple, peeled, cored, and cut into
½-inch-thick slices

1 head butter lettuce

Classic Balsamic Vinaigrette (see page 242)

Season the chicken with salt and pepper. Heat an outdoor grill to medium-high heat or heat a grill pan over medium-high heat. Sear the pineapple for 2 to 3 minutes per side. Make sure you leave the chicken on long enough before you flip so it doesn't stick. Once the chicken is all done, divide the lettuce leaves among four plates and top each with the pineapple, chicken, vinaigrette, and salt and pepper.

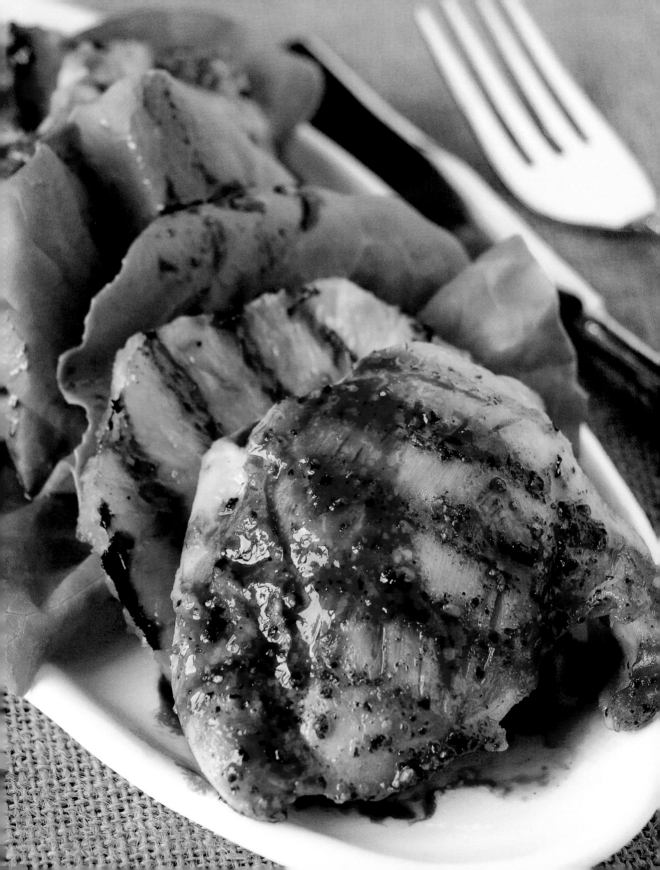

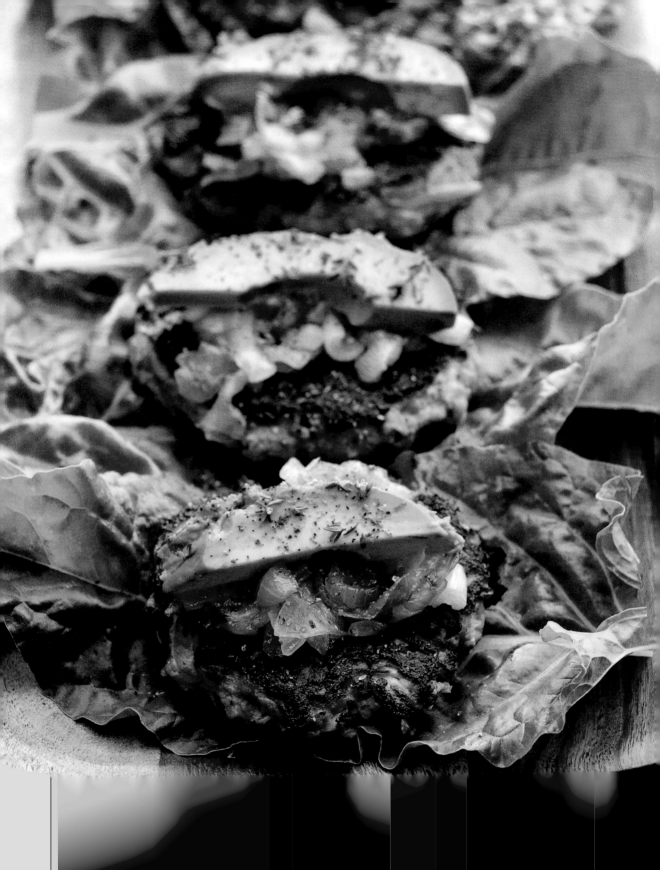

Curry Turkey Burgers with Caramelized Onions

MAKES 8 BURGERS

2 teaspoons ghee

1 large yellow onion, chopped

2 medium carrots, finely grated

1 medium zucchini, coarsely grated

1 pound lean ground turkey

2 tablespoons nutritional yeast

1 large egg

½ teaspoon sea salt

½ teaspoon freshly ground black pepper

1 teaspoon curry powder

1 bunch rainbow chard or 1 head romaine lettuce, washed and dried, leaves intact

In a large pan, melt the ghee over medium heat. Add the onion and cook, stirring occasionally, for 20 to 30 minutes, or until the onion is translucent and very soft. In a large bowl, combine the carrots, zucchini, ground turkey, nutritional yeast, egg, salt, pepper, and curry powder and mix well with your hands. Place another large pan or grill pan over medium heat. Divide the meat mixture into 8 portions and form them into patties. Once the pan is hot, cook the burgers until each side is brown and the burger stays together. Top each burger with caramelized onions and serve wrapped in a large leafy green such as rainbow chard or romaine lettuce.

Skillet Potatoes

SERVES 8

4 Yukon Gold potatoes, cut into ¼-inch-thick slices

3 sweet potatoes, cut into ¼-inch-thick slices

2 tablespoons ghee, melted

2 tablespoons avocado oil

1 teaspoon sea salt

1 teaspoon freshly ground black pepper

1 tablespoon chopped fresh thyme

1 tablespoon chopped fresh rosemary

Preheat the oven to 425°F. In a large bowl, toss the potatoes, ghee, avocado oil, salt, pepper, thyme, and rosemary. Transfer the potatoes to an oven-safe skillet, alternating layers of the Yukon Gold and sweet potatoes. Roast for 1 hour, or until the edges of the potatoes turn brown.

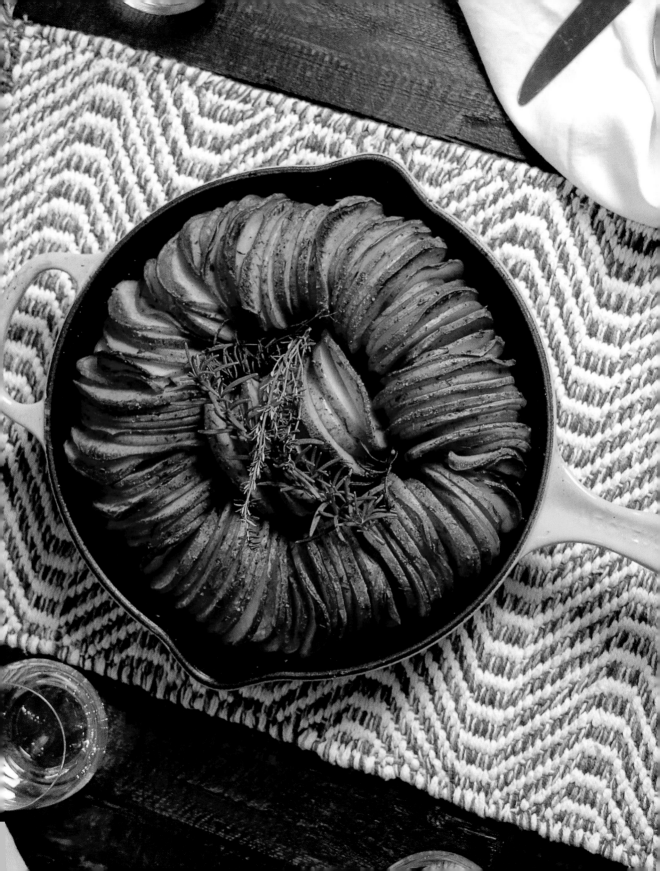

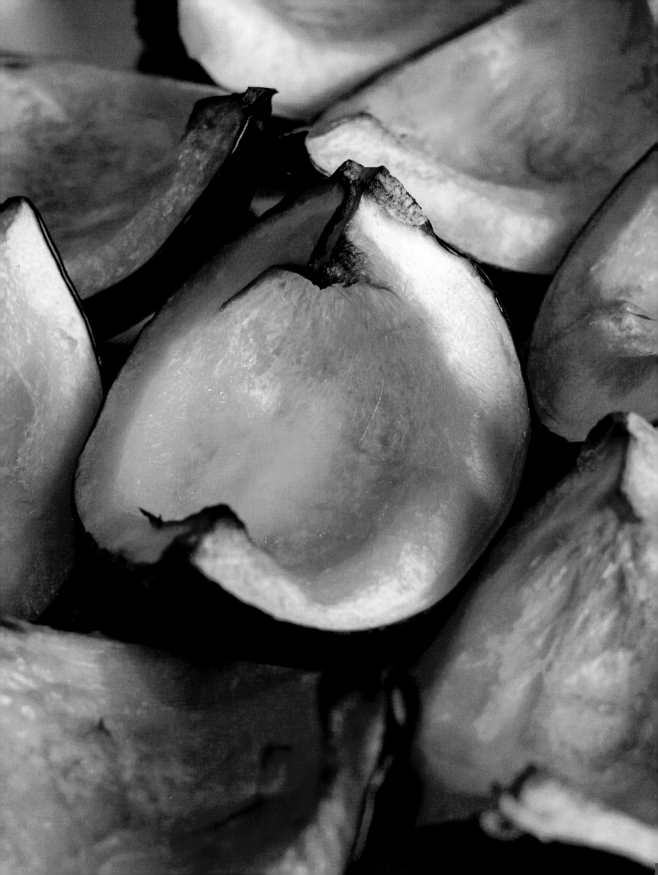

Roasted Acorn Squash

SERVES 8

2 acorn squash, quartered and seeded

1 tablespoon avocado oil

1 tablespoon pure maple syrup

Preheat the oven to 400°F. Rub the squash quarters with the oil and syrup evenly and place on a baking sheet or in a baking dish. Roast for 45 minutes, or until the edges turn brown and you can easily pierce the squash with a fork.

Roasted Butternut Squash

SERVES 6 TO 8

1 butternut squash, peeled, seeded, and cubed

2 tablespoons coconut oil, melted

Preheat the oven to 400°F. Toss the butternut squash with the coconut oil in a bowl. Spread the squash on a baking sheet and roast for 40 to 45 minutes, or until the edges turn brown.

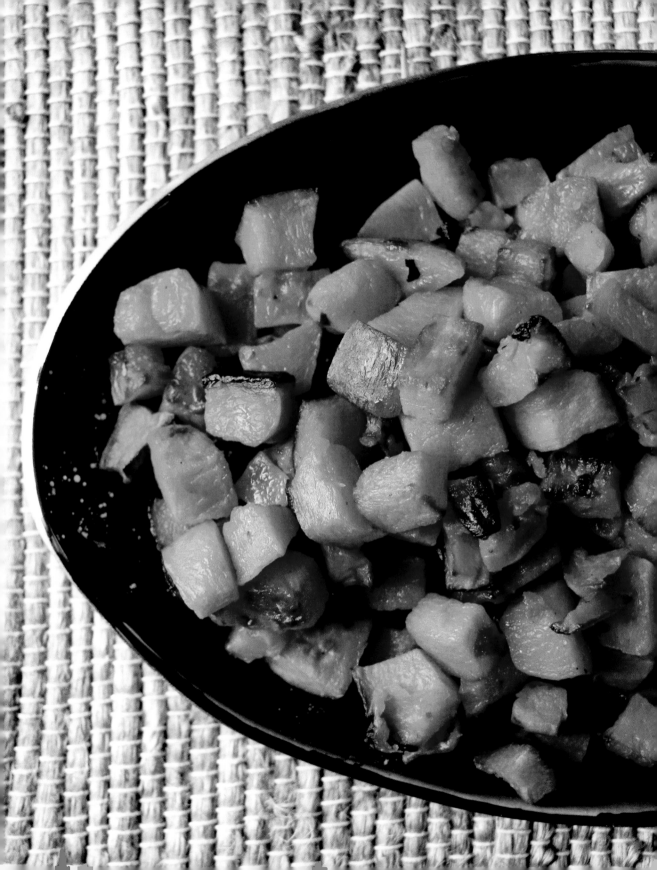

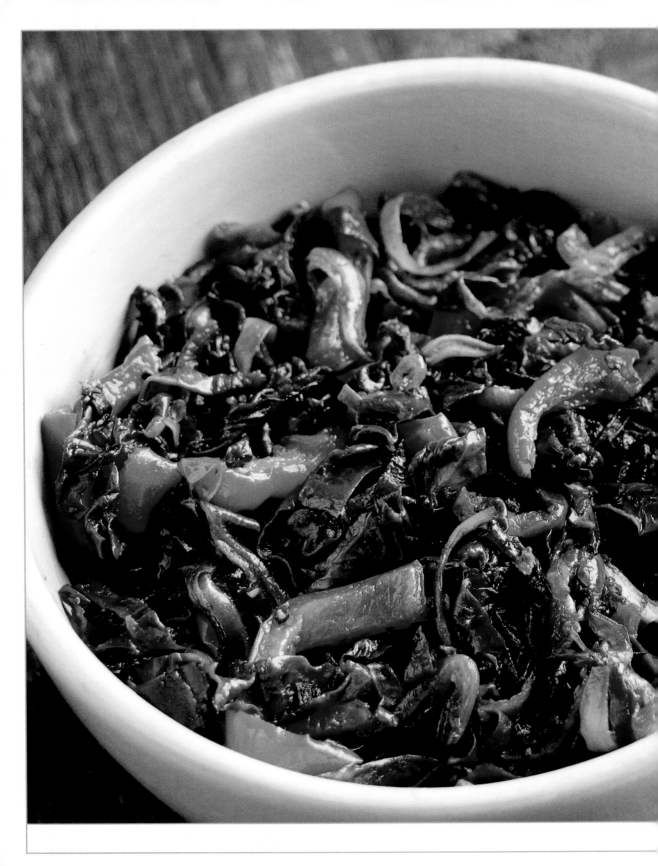

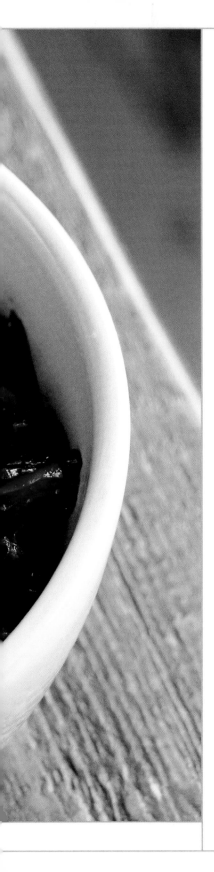

Roasted Purple Cabbage

SERVES 8 TO 10

1 head purple cabbage, shredded

1 large yellow onion, chopped

2 red bell peppers, julienned

2 tablespoons avocado oil

1 teaspoon sea salt

1 teaspoon freshly ground black pepper

Preheat the oven to 400°F. Put the cabbage, onion, peppers, avocado oil, salt, and pepper in a bowl and toss to combine. Divide the mixture between two large baking sheets. Roast for 45 minutes, or until the edges brown, stirring a few times as it cooks.

Kale Salad

SERVES 8 TO 10

½ head purple cabbage, cored and chopped

1 yellow onion, chopped

1 tablespoon avocado oil

1 bunch kale, stemmed, leaves cut into ribbons

½ bunch rainbow chard, stemmed, leaves cut into ribbons

3 tablespoons olive oil

3 tablespoons fresh lemon juice

1 tablespoon coconut aminos

¼ cup pine nuts

2 apples, cored and cubed

Sea salt and freshly ground black pepper

Preheat the oven to 400°F. Toss the cabbage and onion with the avocado oil in a large bowl, then transfer to a baking sheet. Roast for 30 to 40 minutes, or until the vegetables start to turn brown. In another large bowl, massage the kale and chard with the olive oil, lemon juice, and coconut aminos and set aside. Heat a pan over medium heat; lightly toast the pine nuts and set aside. Once the cabbage and onion are finished, let cool, then combine with the massaged greens, pine nuts, and apple. Season with salt and pepper.

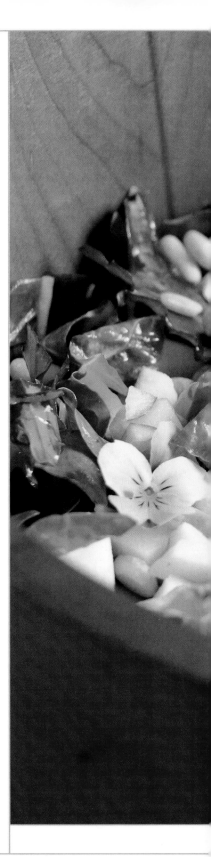

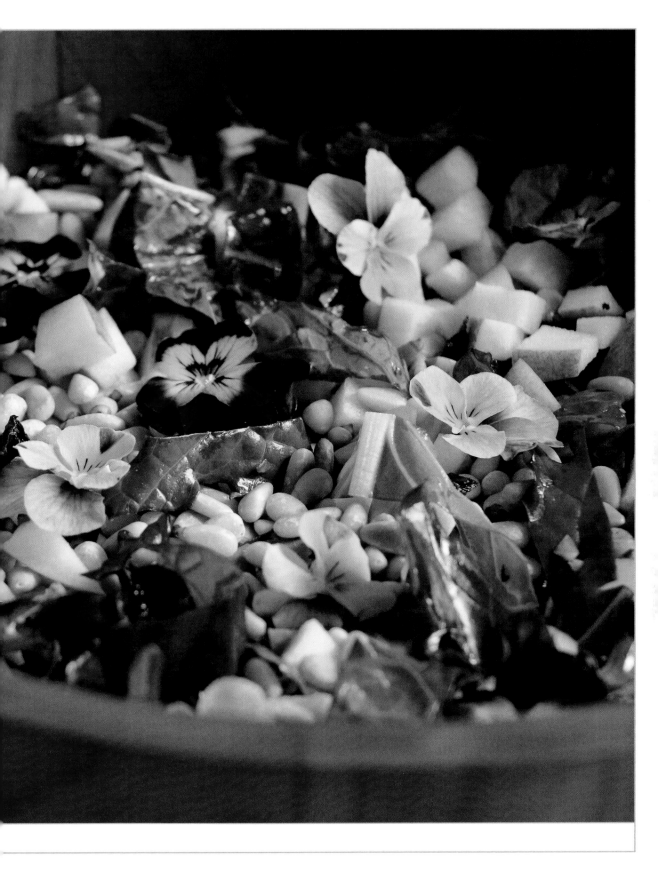

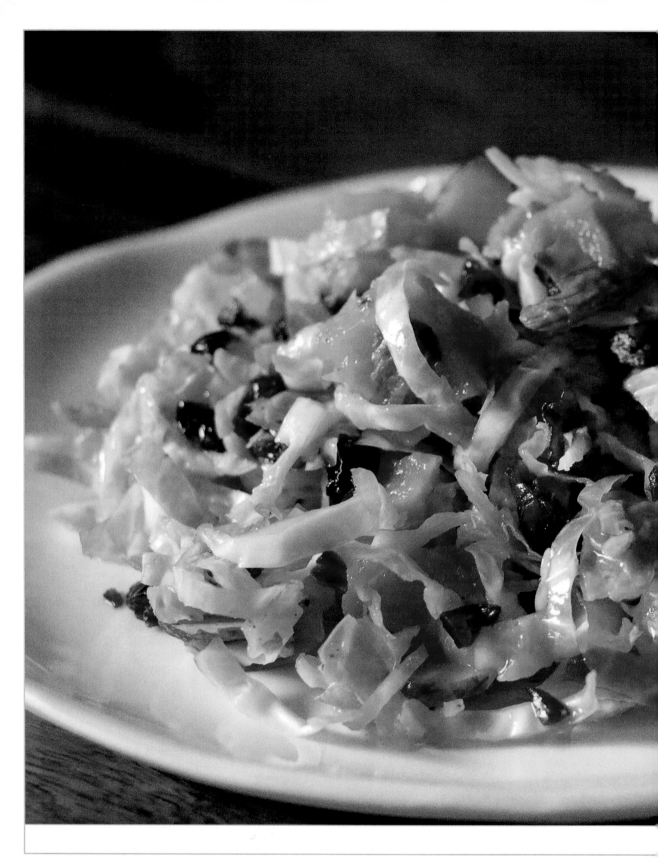

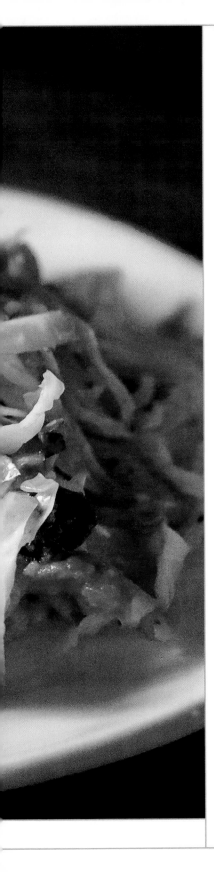

Winter Salad

SERVES 8 TO 10

1 butternut squash, peeled, halved, seeded, and cubed

2 (12-ounce) bags Brussels sprouts, trimmed and shredded

1 cup chopped dried unsweetened cranberries or seeds of 2 pomegranates

1 cup sliced almonds

DRESSING

¼ cup olive oil

Juice of 1½ lemons

2 tablespoons honey

1 tablespoon white wine vinegar

1 tablespoon apple cider vinegar

½ teaspoon sea salt

½ teaspoon freshly ground black pepper

Preheat the oven to 400°F. Put the squash on a baking sheet, cut-side down, and roast for 30 to 40 minutes, or until a fork easily pierces the squash. Remove and let cool. Put the roasted squash, Brussels sprouts, cranberries, and almonds in a large bowl.

Make the dressing: In a small bowl, whisk together all the dressing ingredients. Massage the dressing into the Brussels sprouts.

Bacon-Wrapped Asparagus

SERVES 4

2 bunches asparagus, tough ends trimmed

8 sprigs fresh thyme

4 scallions, sliced lengthwise

8 strips bacon

Freshly ground black pepper

Preheat the oven to 400°F. Divide the asparagus into 8 piles and add a sprig of thyme and half a scallion to each stack. Wrap 1 piece of bacon around each stack. Place the stacks on a baking sheet and roast for 30 minutes or until the bacon browns. Season with pepper before serving.

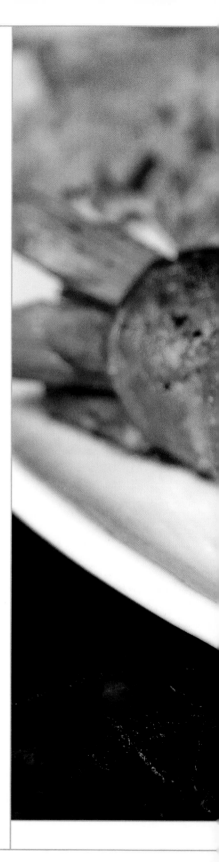

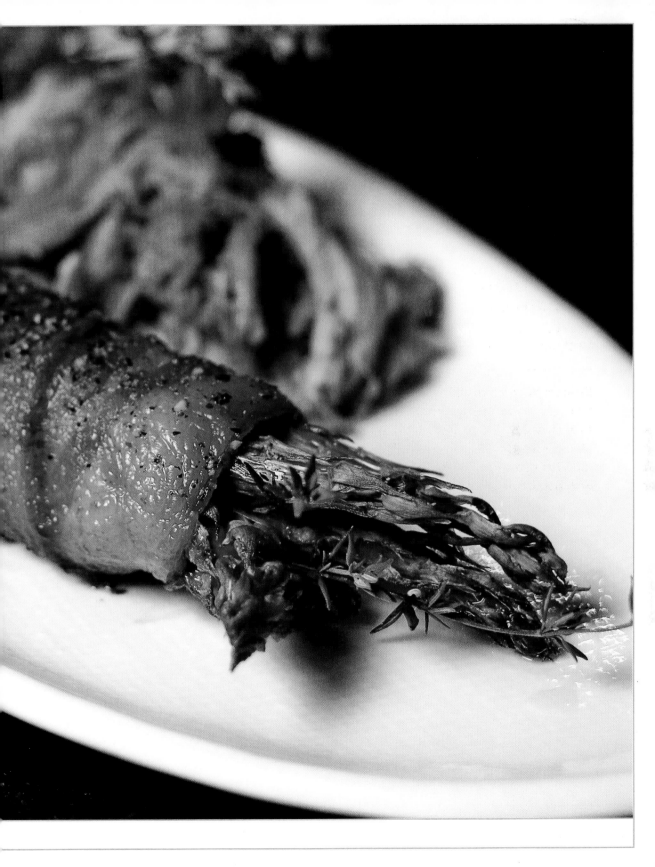

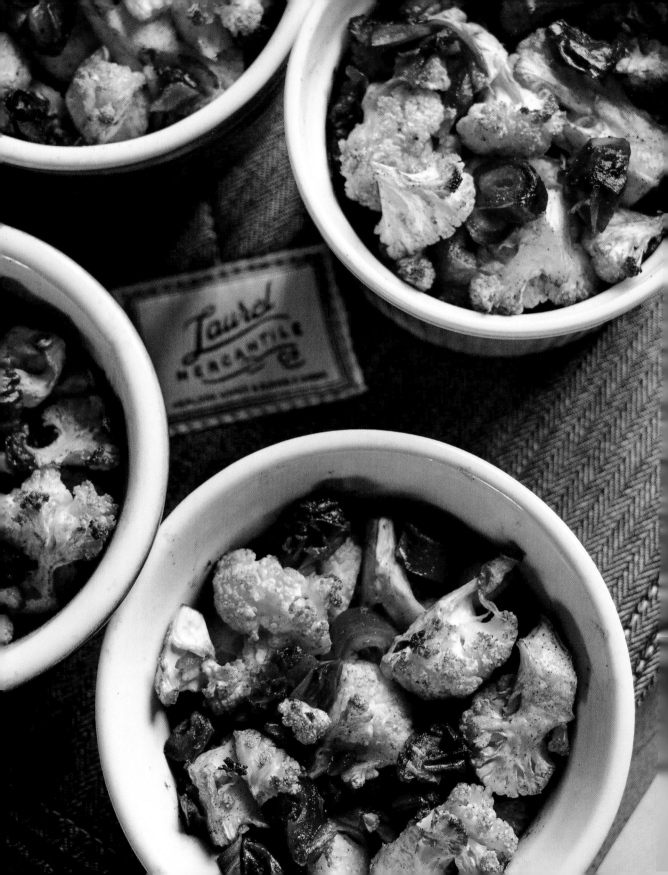

Five-Spice Roasted Cauliflower

SERVES 4

1 head cauliflower, broken into florets

15 pitted dates, chopped

2 tablespoons olive oil

1 teaspoon Chinese five-spice powder

¼ teaspoon sea salt

SAUCE

½ cup tahini

¼ cup hemp seeds

1 teaspoon ground turmeric

¾ teaspoon freshly ground black pepper

Preheat the oven to 400°F. In a large bowl, combine the cauliflower, dates, olive oil, five-spice powder, and salt and toss to combine. Evenly distribute the cauliflower among four small ramekins. Roast for 35 to 40 minutes, or until the tops turn slightly brown.

While the cauliflower roasts, combine all the sauce ingredients in a small bowl and stir until blended. Top the cauliflower with the sauce before serving.

Cast-Iron Skillet Apple Crumble

SERVES 8

APPLES

4 Granny Smith apples, cored and sliced

3 tablespoons ghee, melted

1 teaspoon pure vanilla extract

1 tablespoon ground cinnamon

½ teaspoon ground nutmeg

½ cup coconut sugar

CRUMBLE

¾ cup almond flour

½ cup unsweetened coconut flakes

¾ cup chopped walnuts

½ cup chopped pecans

2 tablespoons chia seeds

1 tablespoon ground cinnamon

2 tablespoons melted coconut oil

2 tablespoons honey

Pinch of sea salt

Preheat the oven to 375°F. **Prepare the apples:** In a large bowl, toss the apples, ghee, vanilla, cinnamon, nutmeg, and coconut sugar to combine. Transfer the mixture to a cast-iron skillet or baking dish.

Make the crumble: Combine the almond flour, coconut flakes, walnuts, pecans, chia seeds, cinnamon, coconut oil, honey and salt in a large bowl and mix well. Spread the crumble on top of the apples. Bake for 35 minutes, or until the crumble starts to turn brown.

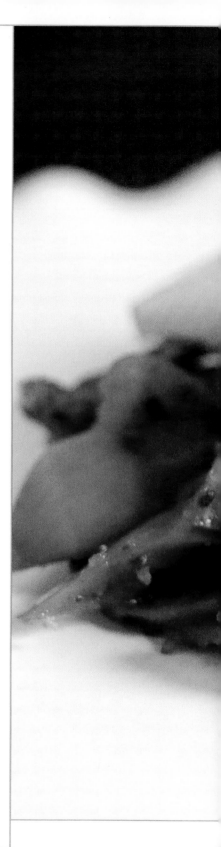

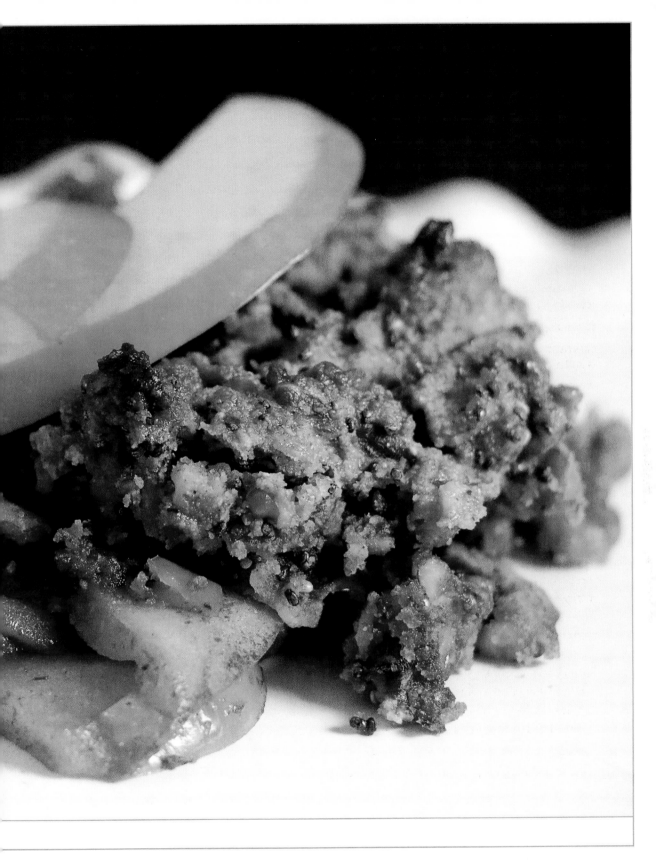

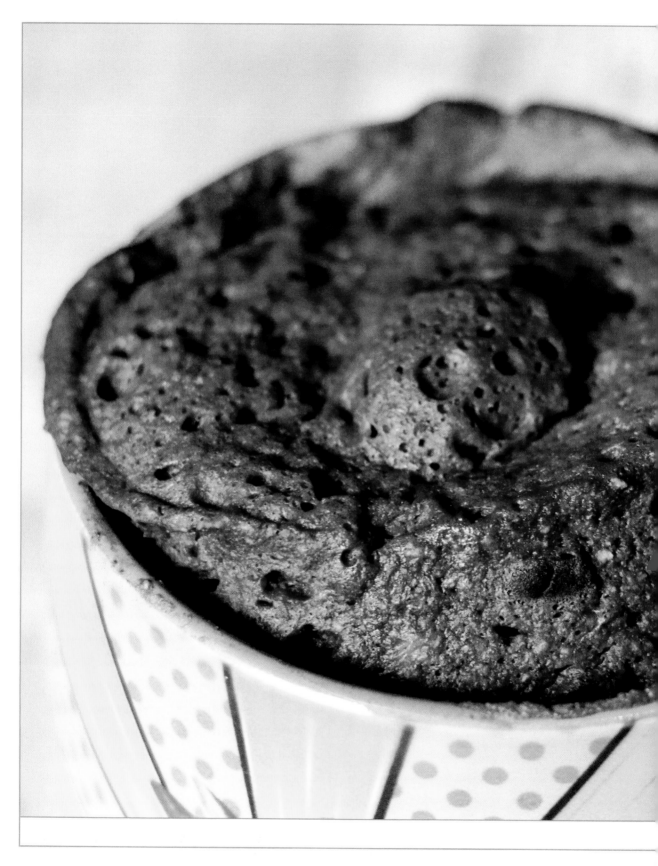

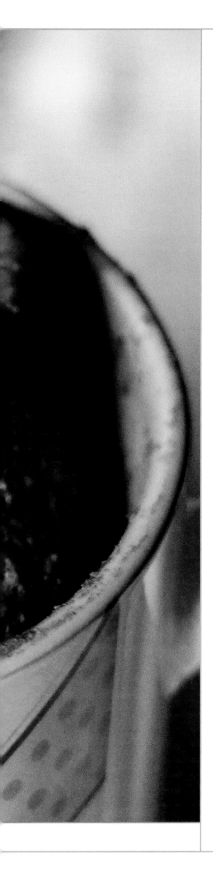

Chocolate Mug Cake

SERVES 1 OR 2

½ banana, plus sliced banana for topping

1 large egg

1 tablespoon unsweetened cocoa powder

1 tablespoon pure maple syrup

2 tablespoons coconut flour

1 tablespoon cocoa nibs, plus more for topping

1 tablespoon semi-sweet chocolate chips

Almond butter, for topping

Honey, for topping

Mash the banana in a coffee mug with a fork. Add the egg, cocoa powder, maple syrup, coconut flour, cocoa nibs, and chocolate chips and stir well. Microwave for 2 minutes, or until the middle of the mixture appears cooked. If sharing, spoon the cake into two bowls (otherwise, just eat it straight from the mug!). Top with almond butter, sliced banana, cocoa nibs, and a drizzle of honey.

Chocolate Chia Pudding

SERVES 2

¼ cup chia seeds

½ cup unsweetened almond milk

2 tablespoons cacao powder

2 tablespoons pure maple syrup

½ cup fresh berries

½ banana, sliced

2 tablespoons cocoa nibs

Combine the chia seeds, almond milk, cacao powder, and maple syrup in a small bowl. Stir and refrigerate for 10 minutes, or until the mixture thickens. Divide between two bowls and serve topped with berries, banana, and cocoa nibs. I often top the dessert with an additional bit of healing herbs such as he shou wu, *Mucuna pruriens*, or triphala.

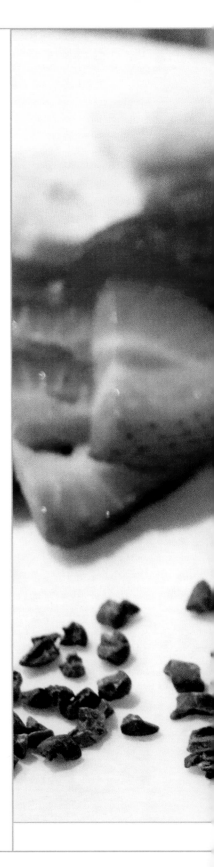

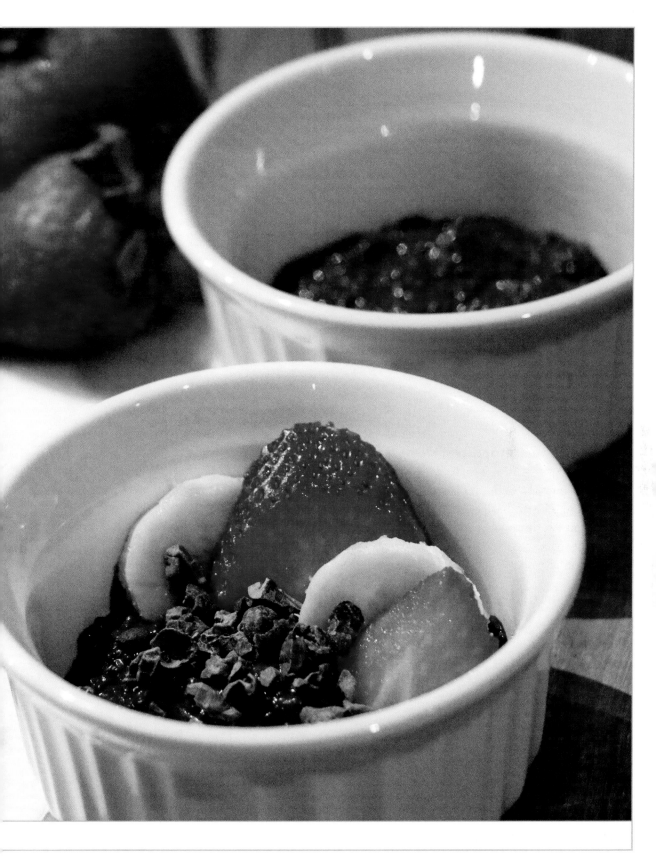

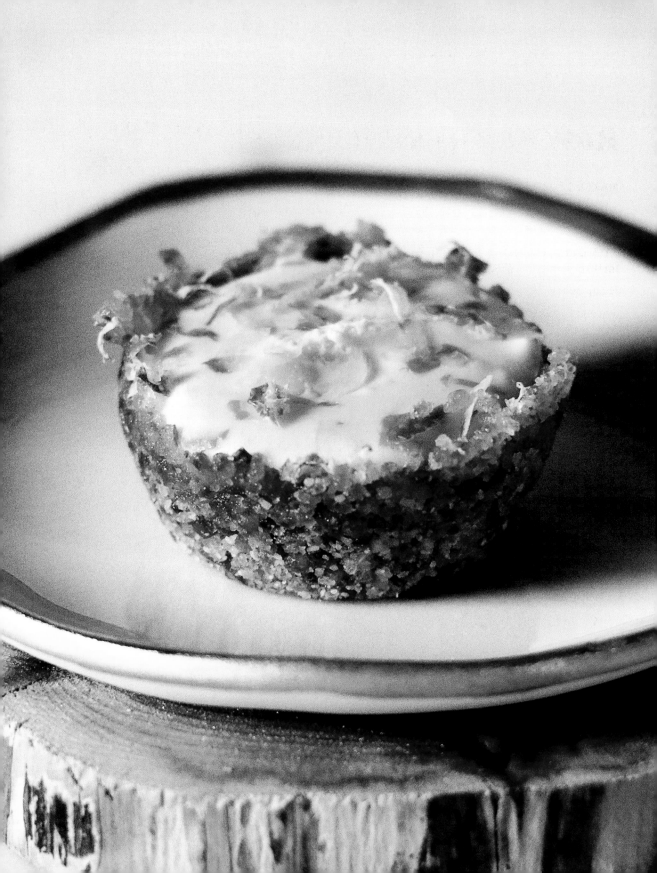

Raw Key Lime Tarts

MAKES 24 TARTS

FILLING

1 (14-ounce) can full-fat coconut milk (solid cream on top only)

¼ cup honey

Juice of 3 limes

CRUST

1 cup pitted dates

1 cup almond flour

1 tablespoon coconut butter, melted

Pinch of sea salt

Zest of 1 lime, for garnish

Make the filling: Scoop out the thick coconut cream from the top of the can of coconut milk and place it in a small bowl (discard the liquid left in the can or save it for another use). Stir in the honey and lime juice and set aside.

Make the crust: In a food processor, combine the dates, almond flour, coconut butter, and salt. Lightly grease two 12-cup cupcake tins. Spoon the crust mixture into the prepared cupcake tins, packing it along the bottom and sides. Spoon the filling evenly into each crust. Top with lime zest. Refrigerate for at least 1 hour, or until the filling firms up before eating. Store any leftovers in the fridge.

Almond Cookies

MAKES ABOUT 12

1 cup almond flour

½ teaspoon baking powder

⅓ cup coconut sugar

Pinch of sea salt

1 tablespoon coconut oil, melted

2 large eggs

⅓ cup unsweetened almond butter

1 teaspoon pure vanilla extract

½ cup semisweet chocolate chips

Preheat the oven to 350°F. Grease a large baking sheet. In a large bowl, combine the almond flour, baking powder, coconut sugar, and salt using a fork. In a separate bowl, combine the coconut oil, eggs, almond butter, and vanilla using a hand mixer. With the mixer running, slowly add the dry ingredients into the almond butter mixture. Mix in the chocolate chips. Using a spoon, scoop the mixture onto the prepared baking sheet and bake for 20 minutes or until slightly brown. Transfer to a wire rack and let cool.

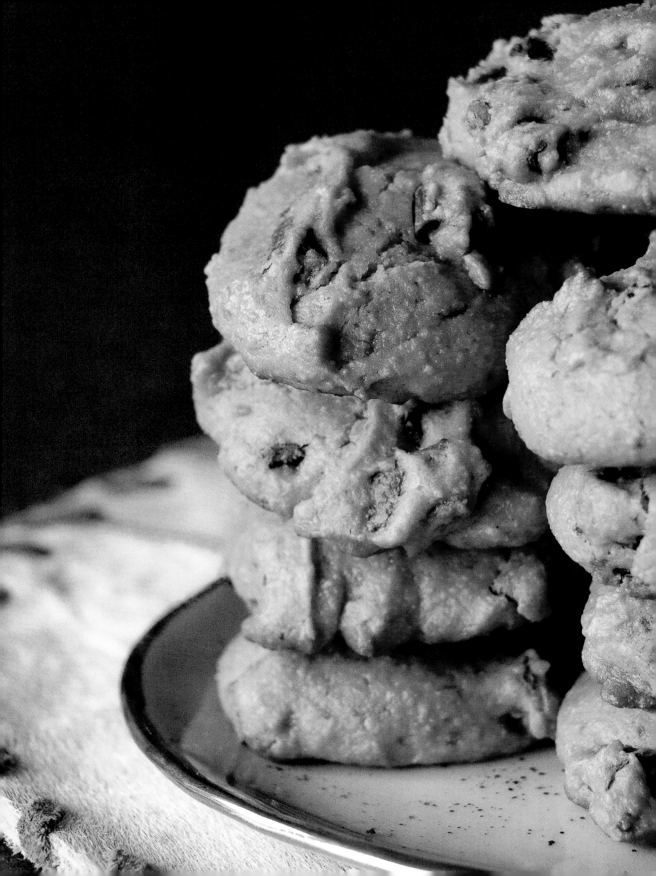

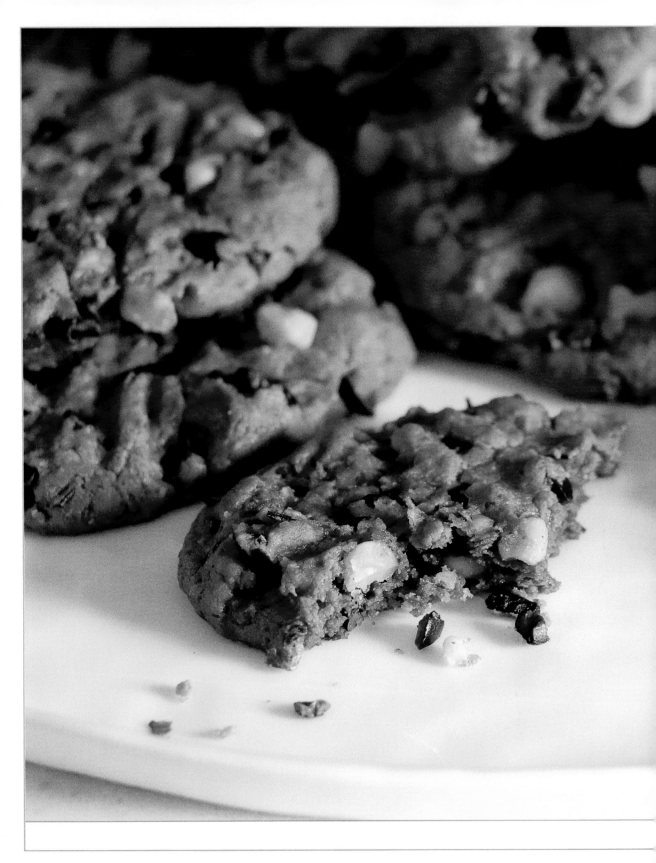

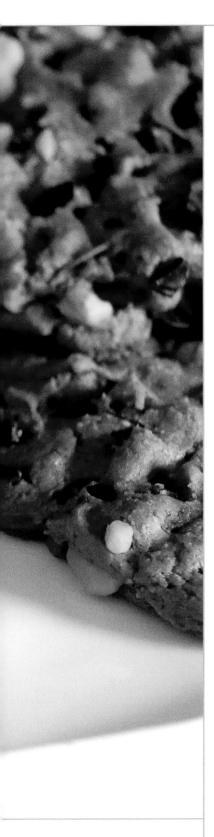

Rosemary Cashew Cookies

MAKES 12 TO 15 COOKIES

1 cup cashew butter

1 cup coconut sugar

1 large egg

½ teaspoon baking soda

1 teaspoon pure vanilla extract

⅛ teaspoon sea salt

½ cup mulberries

½ cup cocoa nibs

½ cup chopped walnuts

1 tablespoon chopped fresh rosemary

Preheat the oven to 350°F. Grease a large baking sheet. In a large bowl using a hand mixer or in the bowl of a stand mixer fitted with the paddle attachment, combine the cashew butter, sugar, egg, baking soda, vanilla, and salt. Beat until smooth, then mix in the mulberries, cocoa nibs, walnuts, and rosemary and continue mixing until evenly distributed. Form the dough into small balls and place them on the prepared baking sheet. Using a fork, press down lightly on each ball to make an X. Bake for 15 to 18 minutes, or until the edges start to brown. Transfer to a wire rack and allow to cool.

Chocolate Chip Peanut Butter Cookies

MAKES 20 SMALL COOKIES

1 cup natural peanut butter (smooth)

¾ cup coconut sugar

1 large egg

½ teaspoon baking soda

1 teaspoon pure vanilla extract

Pinch of sea salt

¾ cup large chocolate chip chunks, or ½ cup regular-size chocolate chips

Preheat the oven to 350°F. Grease a large baking sheet. In a food processor, mix together the peanut butter, coconut sugar, egg, baking soda, vanilla, and salt. Once the mixture is well blended, add the chocolate chips and mix until evenly distributed. Roll the dough into 20 balls, transfer to the prepared baking sheet, and flatten slightly with a fork or spoon. Bake for about 12 minutes, or until the edges brown. Transfer to a wire rack and let cool.

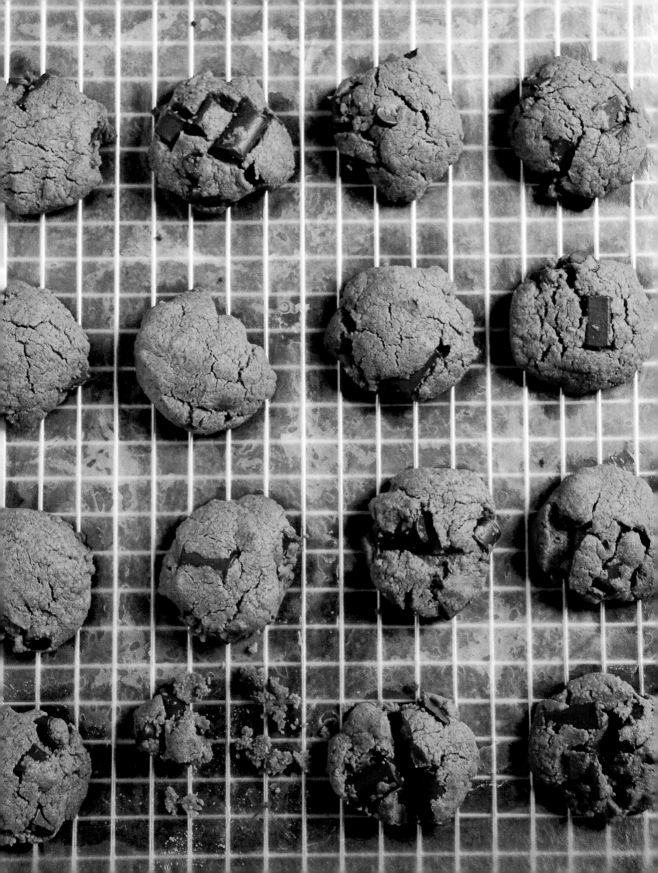

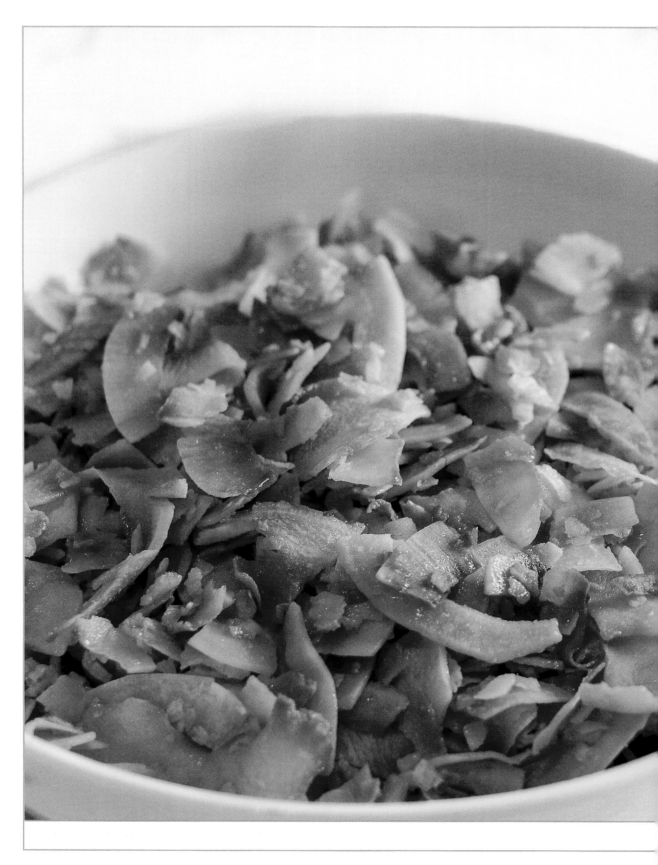

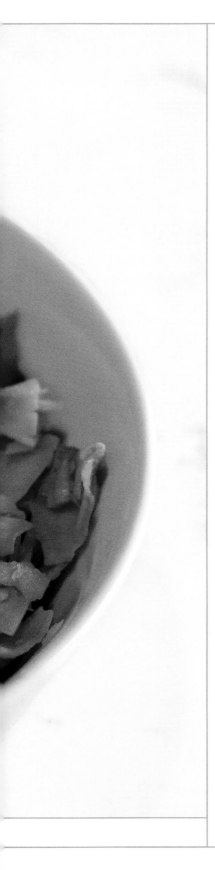

Maple Syrup Coconut Flakes

MAKES 12 TO 14 SERVINGS

1 (7-ounce) bag
unsweetened coconut
flakes

¼ cup pure maple syrup

Preheat the oven to 350ºF. In a large bowl, toss the coconut flakes and syrup. Transfer to a large rimmed baking sheet. Bake for 12 to 15 minutes, stirring once halfway through, or until the flakes turn golden brown

Golden Milk

SERVES 1

1 (1-inch) piece fresh turmeric, grated

1 (1-inch) piece fresh ginger, peeled and grated

1 cup unsweetened almond milk or cashew milk

4 turns of a pepper mill

½ teaspoon ground cinnamon

Pinch of ground cloves

Pinch of ground nutmeg

2 teaspoons honey

In a small saucepan, combine the turmeric, ginger, almond milk, pepper, cinnamon, cloves, and nutmeg and bring just to a boil over medium heat. Remove from the heat and strain into a coffee mug. Drizzle honey on top before serving.

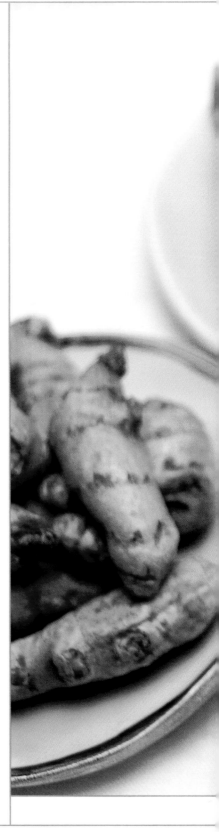

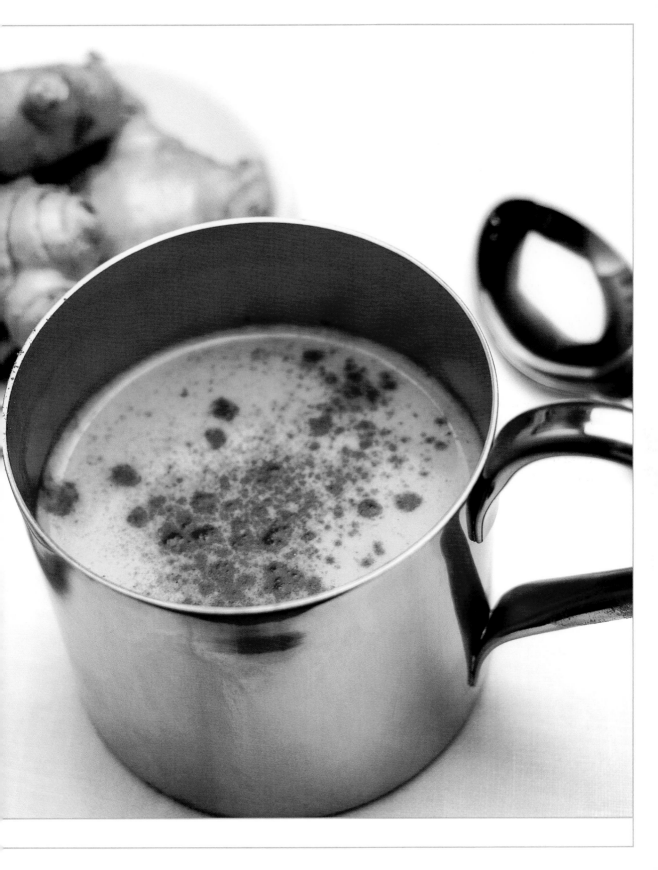

ACKNOWLEDGMENTS

I want to first thank my parents for letting me illegally drive my Mustang Cobra to the local YMCA at the age of fifteen to work out so I could be strong enough to drive my go-kart. Thank you for trusting me.

Thank you to my sister, Brooke, for, of course, being my best friend but also for always being positive and believing in me.

Thank you to my love, Ricky, for putting up with me during the long and exhausting process of writing the workout program, testing all the workouts, writing and editing all the chapters, trying new recipes (especially all the peanut butter cookie ones), and—as a result of then having to wait while I photographed all the food as I went—eating cold food.

Thank you to my business managers, Haley and Allison, for making sure we keep all the facets of Danica Racing in order and for making it as easy as possible for me!

Thank you to Stephen, my coauthor, for putting all of my thoughts, beliefs, theories, and horrible grammar into a legible and comprehensible format. Thank you to Alan, my agent, for making this dream a reality.

Thank you to Megan Newman, my publisher, for believing in me. I believe in my heart this is the first of many helpful and inspiring books.

Thank you to the team at Avery Books—Ashley Tucker, Hannah Steigmeyer, Lindsay Gordon, Anne Kosmoski, Andrea Ho, and everyone who helped make this project a success.

And finally thank you to my #PITribe for taking a chance on a new workout and food program to help me test out *Pretty Intense*. You all made my heart so full from your dedication. I am so proud of you!

INDEX